Diet Cults

Diet Cults

**The Surprising Fallacy at the Core of Nutrition Fads
and a Guide to Healthy Eating for the Rest of Us**

MATT FITZGERALD

PEGASUS BOOKS
NEW YORK LONDON

DIET CULTS

Pegasus Books LLC
80 Broad Street, 5th Floor
New York, NY 10004

Copyright © 2014 by Matt Fitzgerald

First Pegasus Books edition May 2014

Illustrations © 2014 Steve Delmonte

Interior design by Maria Fernandez

Library of Congress Cataloging-in-Publication Data is available.

ISBN: 978-1-60598-560-2

10 9 8 7 6 5 4 3 2 1

Printed in the United States of America
Distributed by W. W. Norton & Company

For Devante

Contents

"It is not what enters into the mouth that defiles the man, but what proceeds out of the mouth, this defiles the man."

Matthew 15:11

Diet Cults

1

Forbidden Fruit

When I was in college I attended a debate between a philosopher and a theologian. The two men squared off over the question of God's existence. The theologian scored a knockout when he got the philosopher to confess his belief in "objective morality" and then delivered a logical proof demonstrating that only God could be the source of objective morality.

The funny thing is that, according to the Bible, morality did not come from God. It came from food. It says so right there in Genesis, on page one, as a matter of fact. We all know the story. The world is newly created, and only one man inhabits it. God plants a special tree in the Garden of Eden and tells Adam, "From any tree of the garden you may eat freely; but from the tree of knowledge of good and evil you shall not eat, for in the day that you eat from it you will surely die." Unfortunately, Adam's wife Eve, who is created immediately after this warning is delivered, falls under the influence of a talking serpent and eats the forbidden fruit, and Adam, choosing loyalty to his wife over obedience to God (as I'd like to think I would have done in his place), eats too. Instantly the couple becomes ashamed of its nakedness, and we've been burdened with consciences—particularly food consciences—ever since.

While the story of the forbidden fruit may be fanciful, I believe that it is substantively accurate. That is to say, I believe that a distinctively human morality really was born from food, through a collision between instinct and language. My historical explanation goes back a little farther than the biblical one, though.

I said "a distinctively human morality" just now because a form of morality exists in many if not most animals. It has been observed, for example, that a hungry lab rat won't eat if eating causes a fellow rat to experience a painful shock. Mother hens are known to mirror the distress of their chicks. The brains of monkeys contain structures that are almost identical to structures in human brains that host our empathetic instincts.

Human morality is undeniably more sophisticated than the proto-morality of other animals, however. Only a human being would leap to his death from a twelfth-floor balcony after photographs in which he is seen dressed in women's underwear are exposed on the Internet, or despise a fellow human being for no reason other than that he believes in a different way of eating.

How did human morality become so much more complex and nuanced than the inborn sense of right and wrong we see in other species? Well, food had a lot to do with it.

The World Is Our Oyster
It all started more than six million years ago, when an ape species similar to the modern chimpanzee underwent an evolutionary

split. One line of descendants changed a little and became our cousin the chimp. The other line changed a lot and became homo sapiens. Scientists believe that the cause of the split was the decision made by some of those primeval apes to venture out of the trees and onto the African savanna. It is suspected that climate change influenced this decision. Specifically, a period of increasing dryness may have caused the savanna to encroach onto jungle territory, shrinking the apes' food supply. The most clever, adaptable, and adventurous apes dropped from the leafy branches to the grassy plains in search of alternative foods—and found them.

The adaptability of these clever apes was paid forward to future generations in the form of evolutionary changes that made them ever more adaptable. Over the span of millions of years, a succession of hominid species descending from the first floor-dwelling primates became increasingly adept at surviving in all kinds of terrestrial environments. Archeological evidence suggests that most of the changes that occurred in the process by which homo sapiens evolved from the earliest hominids generated creatures that were capable of finding, gathering, capturing, killing, cultivating, and domesticating a greater variety of foods. Our species emerged as the master omnivore of planet Earth, capable of extremely diverse eating but also dependent on dietary diversity, both physically and psychologically. We are not koala bears that can blithely thrive on eucalyptus leaves alone.

Above all else it was a large and growing brain that made the succession of species between the proto-chimps of seven million years ago and modern humans increasingly dietetically adaptive. Novel brainpower enabled the hominids of the Paleolithic period to invent tools and techniques that brought more and more foods into their diet. Big brains also furnished them with communication skills that supported sophisticated methods of cooperative food foraging, as well as reasoning skills that were used to make smart dietary choices as new options presented themselves. At least 164,000 years ago, for example, one human gambled on wading into the sea to extract shellfish to eat, and his success added seafood to the diet of the species.

Dietary experimentation is risky, though. Whenever a creature eats something it has never eaten before, there is a chance of disaster. There must have been many a disaster throughout the prehistory and early history of our species as we continually put strange stuff in our mouths to learn whether or not it was good to eat. Consider the example of strychnos nux-vomica, a plant that produces fruit that is attractive, sweetly fragrant, and poisonous, so that our ancestors in Southeast Asia and Australia (where the plant is native) were beguiled into tasting it and met with deadly consequences when they did. Yet the fruit of the strychnos nux-vomica is almost indistinguishable from the bael fruit, which, although terrible-tasting, is nontoxic and even medicinal. As they say, you never know until you try.

The knowledge gained through such experimentation was transmitted from person to person, generation to generation, in the form of rules about eating. Almost from the very beginning, this passing down of collected food lore must have carried a moral element, because even rats have enough inborn conscience to go hungry if eating hurts another rat. As our brains grew larger and our language skills more sophisticated, this moral element intensified.

Distinctively human morality was born—symbolically, anyway—when eating unhealthy food changed from a mere *bad idea* into a *wrongful act*. Among the first recognized crimes was that of eating things *verboten* (a crime that delivered its own penalty as often as those taboo foods were poisonous). Perhaps even older is the crime of feeding forbidden things to others with bad intent, as that talking snake did to poor Eve in the Garden of Eden.

Group identity played a central role in the transformation of eating the wrong foods from a mere mistake into a codified sin.

At some point, gobbling "forbidden fruits" became something that *our kind just doesn't do*. Imagine clan A was the first to discover that a certain berry was harmful to human health in some insidious way. Nearby rival clans B, C, and D had not yet figured it out. If a member of clan A snacked on the taboo berry despite his better knowledge, he bore not only the toxic effects but also the *sin* of having eaten something that defied the identity of clan A as distinct from the identities of clans B, C, and D.

The pressure to not eat what one's group did not want one to eat was so severe that a propensity to make moral judgments based on others' food choices became hardwired into human behavior. Yale psychologist Karen Wynn has shown that babies as young as *three months* express approval of puppets who seem to share their food preferences and also manifestly disapprove of puppets who do not share their food preferences.

As cultures became more advanced, they began to make up dietary rules that served *only* to strengthen group identity and had nothing to do with health. It ceased to matter always whether the berry was healthful or harmful—sometimes you couldn't eat it anyway.

I must admit that I have indulged in a little speculation in the last few paragraphs. There is in fact no record of pre-Bronze-Age "food culture" upon which to base some of the foregoing statements. But my speculations are safe ones, I believe, because the oldest surviving records of food culture provide clear evidence that ancient peoples used food laws to create cultural identity and had been doing so for a long time before these records were created.

The best-known early example of cultural identity formation through food is the kosher diet of the ancient Jews. There are 613 rules of correct living for Jews in the Torah. Many of them are food-related. Anthropologists believe that while some of these food rules had origins in exigencies of health, there was no obvious health benefit associated with most of the taboos, and the greater overall purpose of the rules was undoubtedly to define the Jews as distinct from neighboring peoples. The medieval Jewish philosopher Moses Maimonides pointed out that the famous prohibition against eating "kid boiled in its mother's milk" (which even in his time was interpreted as proscribing the consumption of meat and dairy in the same meal) was originally a prohibition against eating a specific sacrificial dish of rival religions.

The Jewish eating laws constituted what we might call a diet cult. I realize that "cult" is a loaded word, but my intent in using it is not merely to be provocative. I believe that "cult" is the best word to identify a way of eating that is morally based, identity forming, community building, and viewed by its followers as superior to all other ways of eating. The neighbors of the ancient Hebrews had diet cults too. Most if not all ancient peoples did.

In fifth-century B.C.E. China, for example, followers of Confucius observed his numerous mandates concerning the preparation, presentation, and consumption of food, including his commandment that rice be the centerpiece of every meal (as it remains for hundreds of millions of Chinese today). Such identity-forming sets of moral rules for eating made each group different from its neighbors, but more than that, as a general phenomenon, diet cults made humans distinct from the lower animals. Other animals ate rationally, to survive. Humans ate by rules that not only aided their survival but that also separated *sacred* from *profane, us* from *them.*

The natural human tendency to form diet cults is neither good nor bad. But there is a tension inherent in it. The restrictions on dietary freedom upon which each diet cult is based stand in opposition to the natural human desire to eat everything we like. There's a tug-of-war taking place at the deepest level of our nature as eaters. On the one hand the omnivorousness that we came by through evolution drives us to eat freely and widely. On the other hand the wisdom we gained through our often catastrophic adventures in omnivorousness has instilled in us an equally deep-seated impulse to resist certain food temptations and to keep others from eating what we ourselves do not.

This dynamic remains with us today. Although our meals now look rather different from those of our ancient ancestors, and although we talk about food rather differently than they did, the old tug-of-war between our yes-saying impulse to eat what we like and our no-saying impulse to eat by the rules of a special group is as vital as ever. I'm sure you experience this dynamic every day in some fashion. And because this tug-of-war persists, the diet cults remain with us too, as I will amply demonstrate in this book. The rules we make concerning right and wrong ways to eat are still largely moral in nature, and they still have as much to do with separating sacred from profane, us and them, as with keeping us alive.

A Brave New (Food) World

The world has shrunk over the last few centuries. Advancements in transportation and communications have brought the four corners of the globe together, allowing food cultures to cross-pollinate. Traditional ways of eating have mixed and, through admixture, multiplied. There is no longer just one way to eat per culture. Today's eater enjoys great freedom to exercise personal preference in choosing what to eat.

In addition to being more diverse and less culturally and geo-graphically partitioned, our foods are more abundant and easily come by than they used to be. For this reason people now eat less for survival and more for pleasure than they did before. Food producers—most of which today are large corporations—work hard to satisfy and to further stoke demand for pleasurable eating experiences. Meanwhile our chefs have elevated the art of cooking to new heights of deliciousness. These several factors have con-spired to unleash our impulse toward unrestricted eating to a degree that was never possible in the past. As a result, pleasure eating has become one of the major diet cults of the modern world.

There are two sub-cults within the cult of pleasure eaters: the fat-salt-sweets (as I call them) and the foodies. Members of both groups—like members of all diet cults—strongly identify with their way of eating and regard it as superior to other ways. Fat-salt-sweets are people who live principally on fast food, snack chips, soft drinks, processed meats, sugary breakfast cereals, and other so-called junk foods. Such people often express disdain for other foods. They may turn down an invitation to eat sushi on the grounds that sushi is not "real food," or proudly assert that Diet Coke is the only thing they ever drink.

The foodies, in turn, look down their noses at the fat-salt-sweets. Some of the most pretentious foodies go so far as to deny they like the taste of fast food. The less pretentious ones merely contend that fine cookery tastes good in a sophisticated way, whereas junk food tastes good in a crude way. There's nothing wrong with a good burger every now and again, they concede, but a truly refined palate will always prefer coq-au-vin to greasy drive-thru fried chicken.

It is interesting to note that pleasure eaters of both types tend to eat more or less the same way their parents did. The group to which a person belongs defines his tastes more than a person's tastes define the group to which he belongs. Even those who do not follow any explicit cultural rules of eating obey implicit rules set by their social environment. The lion's share of our modern dietary freedom of choice goes unused.

Lifelong fat-salt-sweets frequently pay a heavy price for their unrestrained pleasure eating. That cost is exacted in the form of familiar health consequences which include getting fat, looking terrible, being woefully out of shape, aging quickly, becoming diabetic, developing heart disease, and dying young. The foodie's diet is typically healthier than the fat-salt-sweet's, but among the gourmands there are more than a few gluttons who get every bit as fat as the junk-food gobblers do. Indeed, a number of prominent foodies with television cooking shows could stand to lose a few pounds.

The health consequences associated with unfettered pursuit of pleasure in food have inspired new dietary restrictions. A cult of healthy eating has sprung up in counterpoint to the cult of pleasure eating. Of course, rules for healthy eating have existed as long as any rules for eating have existed, but the cult of healthy eating is something relatively new. It did not emerge until the old, ethnically based diet cults had faded away and the health consequences of pleasure eating had become manifest.

This modern cult of healthy eating is made up of innumerable sub-cults that are constantly vying for superiority. A competitive marketplace of healthy diets emerged in the nineteenth century and has been growing ever since. Like consumer products in commercial markets, each of these diets has a brand name and is advertised as being better than competing brands.

The recruiting programs of the healthy-diet cults consist almost entirely of efforts to convince prospective followers that their diet is the One True Way to eat for maximum physical health. Advocates of each cult cite scientific evidence to support their claims of superiority. This tactic is necessary because in the modern world, science has displaced religious and cultural tradition as the recognized authority for all health-related truth claims. So vegetarians, for example, say that theirs is the healthiest way to eat because science has proven that animal foods cause heart disease and other health problems. Meanwhile, low-carb diet advocates say that theirs is the healthiest way to eat because carbohydrates are scientifically proven to cause obesity and diabetes. Not to be outdone, proponents of the Paleo Diet say that, according to evolutionary logic, all foods that entered the human diet after our days as hunter-gatherers—including grains, dairy, and legumes—are bad for us. And so forth.

Now, if science really had proven conclusively that there was only one clearly defined healthy way to eat, or that a particular diet was indisputably the healthiest, then the competitive marketplace of healthy-diet cults that we are surrounded by would not exist. But science has *not* identified the healthiest way to eat. In fact, it has come as close as possible (because you can't prove a negative) to confirming that *there is no such thing as the healthiest diet.* To the contrary, science has established quite definitively that humans are able to thrive equally well on a variety of diets. Adaptability is the hallmark of man as eater. For us, many diets are *good* while none is *perfect.*

This consensus belief of the nutrition science mainstream is neatly summarized in the book *What To Eat,* authored by Marion Nestle, one of the most prominent nutrition scientists of her generation. Nestle wrote, "The range of healthful nutrient intake is broad and foods from the earth, tree, or animal can be combined in a seemingly infinite number of ways to create diets that meet health goals."

Having arrived at this conclusion, the nutrition-science mainstream offers guidelines for healthy eating that are more flexible than those of the healthy-diet cults. Originating in big epidemiological studies and validated in major scientific reviews, these guidelines are delivered to the public through a variety of resources, including registered dietitians, community nutrition education programs, a few popular books like Marion Nestle's, and the USDA's MyPlate system. They consist mainly of basic recommendations concerning how often to eat various types of foods. Many of the recommendations are familiar to you: eat at least five servings of fruits and vegetables daily, eat whole grains instead of refined grains, eat fish at least twice a week, avoid sugary drinks, and so forth. Although quite specific, these standards are loose enough so that twenty people with twenty different sets of food preferences (and budgets) could follow the guidelines faithfully and yet eat in twenty distinct ways, whereas the healthy-diet cults demand a greater degree of conformity.

How is it that the leaders of healthy-diet cults and their followers are able to believe that their way of eating is the One True Way when the nutrition-science mainstream says so emphatically that there is no such thing? The short answer is that people believe what they want to believe. The complete answer is that people want to believe that a certain way of eating is the best way because it gives them a sense of identity and a feeling of belonging. It's the work of that old, no-saying human impulse to eat according to the rules of a special group, which is often much stronger than the reasoning faculties.

While all of the healthy-diet cults are based on false doctrine, most of them are able to deliver the results that their followers seek. What makes them effective is not the truth of their supporting doctrine but their special appeal to the "diet-cult instinct" in human nature. Eating healthfully is not easy in the modern world. The yes-saying impulse to eat for pleasure is powerful, and indulging that instinct has never been easier. Most people put up little resistance against it. A high level of motivation is needed to swim against the tide, saying "no" to "bad" food and "yes" to "good" food. The healthy-diet cults supply this motivation by appealing to the opposing impulse, our instinctual desire to belong to a group of people defined by a strict way of eating.

For all their talk about science, the diet cults don't really win new members by appealing to their reason. They grab people by the heart—or by the gut, as it were. We are conditioned to think of healthy eating as a rational choice. Step one: the benefits are explained to us. Step two: we are convinced of the benefits. Step three: we make a rational decision to begin practicing the healthy-eating philosophy that promises those benefits. But it doesn't really work that way. The choice to eat healthily is not made logically. It's about *identifying* with a healthy way of eating.

That old no-saying impulse makes each of us potentially receptive to the idea that a certain rule-bound way of eating is the One True Way. If we just give in and embrace the doctrine of a particular cult, then suddenly it seems so much easier to escape the path of pleasure eating and begin walking along a new path of eating "right" that is made smooth by our belief in the godlike perfection of the system, and by a feeling of superiority we gain over dietary infidels, not to mention the camaraderie of our fellow cult members.

The specific cult whose "science"-backed shtick a person finds most convincing usually depends on his or her identity biases. I know a fellow named Richard who became a vegan when he was forty years old. Previously he had been an abject pleasure eater. Veganism has existed a lot longer than nutrition science has existed. Its origins are not scientific but spiritual. Only fairly recently have vegans started justifying their way of eating on scientific grounds. My friend Richard did a lot of reading on the science of veganism and came away believing that veganism was the correct way to eat. But this happened only *after* he had already given up animal foods. And, of course, he cherry-picked his sources, ignoring experts like Walter Willett at the Harvard School of Public Health and going straight to gurus like Caldwell Esselstyn, a man who could never get a job at the Harvard School of Public Health. The nutrition-science mainstream does not believe it is necessary to go vegan to attain maximum health. The real reason Richard became a vegan was that he was a man of extremes (a successful entrepreneur, a recovered alcoholic) and he knew that in order to successfully leave behind his bad eating habits, he had to choose an extreme alternative. The extremism of veganism appealed to his personality.

What is true for veganism and for Richard is true in some measure for all healthy-diet cults and for all of their followers. Scientific justifications and rational persuasion are mere covers for the identity-based forces that truly govern the conversion process. It feels good to believe in something.

Agnostic Healthy Eating

Chances are you're neither a fully committed follower of the cult of pleasure eating who cares nothing about nutrition nor a card-carrying member of any healthy-diet cult. You're probably reading this book because you want to eat more healthfully than you do. If so, you're hardly alone. One reason so many of us get stuck in a rut of eating less wholesomely than we mean to is that some of the least healthy foods are among the most tempting and ubiquitous. In a world without potato chips, it would be easier for many of us to eat more broccoli.

That's not the only problem, however. Another issue is that, collectively, the healthy-diet cults have at least halfway convinced all of us that it is impossible to attain maximum health without joining a diet cult. While on some level we may recognize that mainstream scientific guidelines for healthy eating like those that are embodied in MyPlate will do the job, we don't really embrace these guidelines as a viable alternative to the diet cults. That's largely because there is no community of "agnostic healthy eaters" that we who have a hard time swallowing the dogma of any particular cult can identify with and join. Instead, we are left to discover this way of eating for ourselves, which is not easy given the noise you'll be exposed to if you Google "healthy diet."

Agnostic healthy eaters do exist, but they are mostly invisible. The nearest thing to a community of agnostic healthy eaters I've encountered is the community of professional endurance athletes. Lucky for me, I meet these people often in my work as an endurance sports writer, coach, and nutritionist. By studying the eating habits of world-class cyclists, runners, and triathletes I have learned that while most of them maintain very healthy diets, very few belong to diet cults. They simply eat as the dietary guidelines based on mainstream nutrition science would have them eat, which is to say they eat *everything*, but they eat a lot more of the healthiest foods (such as vegetables) than they do of the least healthy foods (such as soft drinks). An athlete myself—as well as a dietary skeptic who has always been turned off by the diet cults—I eat this way too, and promote it among recreational athletes through my writing and speaking.

Professional endurance athletes have somewhat different motivations for eating healthily than others do. Racers eat to win. They will gladly do whatever is required dietetically to maximize their fitness and performance. But at the same time they are resistant to any dietary restrictions that are not relevant to their goals. Unlike those who join the healthy-diet cults, competitive endurance athletes do not need the special motivation that is supplied by weird restrictions. The desire to win supplies all the motivation they need. If they could win races as pure pleasure eaters—either fat-salt-sweets or foodies—many of them would. On the other hand, if they had to eat in some super-restrictive way to win—for example, getting exactly 16.5 percent of their calories from protein and avoiding all foods whose names start with the letter "M"—they would do that just as readily.

What elite endurance athletes truly desire is *the least restrictive diet that is sufficient to yield maximum fitness and performance.* And they've found it. Decades of trial and error undertaken by athletes around the world have revealed that agnostic healthy eating—a flexible, inclusive diet consistent with mainstream nutrition-science guidelines—is sufficient to support maximum fitness and performance. The tighter restrictions of the healthy-diet cults are not necessary. In fact, they only make it harder for many athletes to maintain healthy eating habits because they drain too much of the pleasure out of eating.

As a group, top endurance athletes are, I believe, the healthiest people in the world. They owe their supreme health as much to exercise as they do to diet. But even so, they are living proof that a flexible and inclusive kind of healthy diet is good enough to support not only maximum fitness and athletic performance but also the highest degree of all-around *health* that is attainable.

Wouldn't you like to feel as robust and vital, function as well (in everyday life, if not on the racecourse), and be as happy with how you look as these athletes? I'm sure you would. And you can—but you must eat better. You do not, however, have to join a diet cult. As I've said, most of the healthy-diet cults work well. But they're nonstarters for many people—too doctrinaire, too restrictive, too . . . cultish. People like us cannot sustain super-healthy eating if doing so forces us to sacrifice our reason and deny our natural omnivorousness.

Olympic runners and their sporting cousins show us that it is possible to eat a basically "normal" diet and yet look and feel spectacular. There are other agnostic healthy eaters besides endurance athletes, but not as many as there ought to be. The challenge for those of us whose livelihood does not depend on winning races is that we lack a motivation to eat healthily that makes up for our inability to identify with any of the healthy-diet cults. The best alternative source for such motivation, and the only one that can work on a mass scale, is a visible community of agnostic healthy eaters that is always welcoming in more rational, independent eaters like us. The purpose of this book is to initiate the process of creating a thriving community of agnostic healthy eaters that makes this way of attaining maximum health a realistic alternative to the diet cults for more people—starting with you.

The Journey Ahead

Two things must happen if my vision is to become a reality. First, a great many people must recognize that all of the healthy-diet cults are fundamentally the same—founded upon the same mythology—and must reject them collectively. We need to get to a point where diet-cult sales pitches of all kinds are easily identified as such and shot down with the words, "Oh, dear, I see they've gotten to you too." The object is not to make the community of agnostic healthy eaters as insufferably smug as the healthy-diet cults often are, but rather to instill a certain degree of us-and-them pride in our group, because that old no-saying dietary impulse exists in us too, so we might as well use it.

The second thing that needs to happen is that the agnostic healthy-eating alternative must be well defined so that it's easy to follow.

Curing folks of subtle diet-cult brainwashing is a harder job than defining agnostic healthy eating, so the first of these matters will occupy most of our attention in these pages. Even those of us who stand outside the healthy-diet cults have been infected by them to some degree. There is an underlying creed shared by all of the healthy-diet cults that is based on a number of unquestioned articles of faith. Each of us has been exposed to these myths so frequently that we have been influenced by them despite our rejection of the particulars of each cult's doctrine. These shared myths include the belief that human nutrition is perfectible, the notion that some foods and nutrients are absolutely bad, others absolutely good, and the assumption that diet is relevant only to *physical* health. My goal in the next thirteen chapters is to reverse all this brainwashing. You may not require as much deprogramming as others do, but we will take our time in deconstructing the mythology of the healthy-diet cults. For it is our shared experience of this journey that will bind us together as a community of agnostic healthy eaters. Therefore we mustn't rush.

The myth-busting mission we're set to embark upon is perhaps a little different from what you might be expecting from a book called *Diet Cults*: namely, a breezy survey of popular diets that discredits each one's claims of superiority. While our project will require some such discrediting, it will be done only as a means to a greater end. Frankly, the debunking is mostly old news. With help from the popular media, science has done a good job of exposing the faults in, and limitations of, many popular diets. The problem is that this process hasn't led anywhere. Proving that an individual diet is not the One True Way still leaves open the possibility that another diet is. I want to go deeper and show that all diets that claim to be the healthiest are based on the same false assumptions—that these diets are, in fact, *diet cults*. My aim is to create a kind of "class consciousness" among those of us who earnestly desire to attain a level of health that can be attained only through very careful eating and who have rejected the cults.

In the pages ahead, we will travel across the planet and through time to encounter true stories and real histories that, when viewed through the lens of current science, expose the speciousness of things we have been coaxed to believe about nutrition and diet. As these examples pile up, the whole mythology on which the diet cults are collectively based will come crumbling down. My hope is that when this journey is concluded, you will know what I know: that you can attain maximum health through a diet that is flexible, inclusive, and rational. I hope too that you will be left eager to pursue this approach to eating.

In the book's final chapter, I will share concrete guidelines for agnostic healthy eating. I say "guidelines," but there is exactly one rule, which I created originally for endurance athletes but is relevant to everyone. There are ten basic types of food, which can be sensibly ranked in order of quality. My one rule of agnostic healthy eating *requires* that you eat just enough of the higher quality food types, such as vegetables, and *allows* you to consume just enough of the lower quality food types, such as sweets, to support maximum health. While fully consistent with mainstream nutrition-science recommendations like those of MyPlate, this agnostic healthy-eating game is simpler, more systematic, and therefore easier to practice.

But wait: Is this agnostic healthy eating game not just another diet cult? No. For I do not claim that agnostic eating is the One True Way. I claim only that you will find agnostic healthy eating to be the easiest way to eat for maximum health if you're turned off by diets that claim to be the One True Way. What's more, unlike diet-cult dogma, this rule allows all kinds of flexibility to practice agnostic healthy eating your way, which may not be my way.

The last thing I'm trying to do here is to recruit followers. I leave that to the diet-cult gurus. It is comrades that I seek. Like that great skeptic and careful eater Friedrich Nietzsche, whom we'll meet again before our journey is complete, "I need living companions who will follow me because they want to follow themselves."

2

100 Foods to Eat Before You Die

Thomas Jefferson, third president of the United States of America, was a celebrated epicure. The frequent dinners hosted at the White House during Jefferson's tenure as head of state were legendary, his invitations highly coveted. His hand-picked chef, French expatriate Honoré Julien, was tasked to create meals of great variety and supreme quality for the president and his lofty guests. No fewer than ten dishes were served at a typical gathering: soup to start and then perhaps fish, beef, ham, mutton, veal, fried eggs, assorted vegetables, desserts ranging from custards and ice cream to fruit and cheese, and to drink: wine, cider, and malt liquor.

Present at many of these dinners was Jefferson's personal secretary, a capable outdoorsman and army officer named

Meriwether Lewis. On June 20, 1803, Jefferson penned a letter to Lewis in which the lieutenant was instructed to lead the first expedition across the continent of North America on behalf of the U.S. Government. Lewis spent the next eleven months in feverish preparation for the journey, and he put more time and effort into preparing to feed the expedition than he put into any other part of it.

Lewis was right to obsess over the problem of keeping a couple of dozen travelers fed for at least one year, maybe two, as they made a transcontinental trek of some five thousand round-trip miles through alien wilderness. It's not as if they could pull up to a fast-food restaurant drive-thru window at any given freeway exit. The nearest thing they could count on—*maybe* count on—was trade with the Native Americans they would encounter along the way. To that end, Lewis was sure to include among the supplies he ordered for the expedition a vast quantity of colored beads and other gewgaws that the indigenes were said to covet. But he knew that exchanging beads for pemmican could not alone save his men from starvation in even the rosiest scenario. So Lewis also packed piles of firearms and plenty of gunpowder and shells for hunting (as well as for protection against Indians not amenable to trade). White men knew precious little about the flora and fauna of the deep interior at that time (gathering such knowledge was one of the objectives of the mission). But the prevailing belief was that the West was teeming with game, and Lewis trusted that fresh meat would be one of the most reliable sources of calories for the "Corps of Discovery," as it was officially known.

Like Indian trade, however, hunting in unknown territory was a prospect in which Lewis could not afford to invest blind trust. The party would have to carry some lasting form of nourishment—not too much, lest its progress be impeded, but enough to see the men through emergencies. Transporting food was easier said than done in the early nineteenth century. Food storage and preservation methods were only slightly more advanced than they had been a couple of thousand years before. If the expedition had started only a decade later, the Corps of Discovery would have benefited from canning and bottling, technologies that did not exist in 1804. As it was, they had to rely on many of the same tools and practices that were used to feed the armies of Alexander the Great.

In his research into portable rations, Lewis discovered dried soup. He thought it ingenious. Meats were boiled down to a thick broth, dried, and cut into cakes that were packed into tin cans. When needed, the soup was reconstituted with boiling water. As long as it was kept dry in the interim, this ration of last resort remained usable for many months. Lewis ordered 193 pounds of dried soup for the expedition.

When Lewis set out from Pittsburgh with eleven men (William Clark and the rest of the party would join them in St. Louis) on August 31, 1803, he did not really know what the Corps would eat through most of the voyage. Yet he was confident that adequate nourishment would be obtained, even if many of the foods that provided this nourishment were unfamiliar. Such confidence rested on Lewis's understanding of a basic fact of human nutrition: people can eat an incredible variety of things.

On the surface, the great feasts that Meriwether Lewis had enjoyed at the table of Thomas Jefferson and the very different ways of eating the lieutenant (now captain) would experience during the two-year expedition he undertook at the president's behest were totally different. But on a deeper level they were much the same. Jefferson included dozens of species of plants and animals (among other edible things, such as honey and mushrooms) in his dinners. He did so because people enjoy variety in their eating. People enjoy variety in their eating because human beings have a long history of omnivorousness. And we have a long history of omnivorousness partly because we are a species of explorers, of men like Meriwether Lewis, and have been since we first left the trees.

The men of the Corps of Discovery indeed ate an incredible variety of things during their expedition. In her delightful book, *Feasting and Fasting with Lewis & Clark*, Leandra Zim Holland compiled as complete a list as possible of everything the Corps ate and drank during the expedition. There are 242 items on that list. The variety of meats alone is staggering. Holland's list includes (in alphabetical order) antelope, badger, beaver, bear, bighorn sheep, bison, brant, cormorant, coyote, crow, deer, dog, duck, eagle, elk, fox, goose, grouse, hawk, horse, otter, panther, pigeon, plover, porcupine, prairie dog, rabbit, squirrel, turkey, and wolf.

A few years ago, a game called "100 Foods to Eat Before You Die" circulated on Facebook. It was a game that no species other than humans would have thought to play. The format was simple. Players were presented with a list of 100 mostly exotic foods (chitterlings, eel, fois gras, haggis, sea urchin) from all parts of the world and were instructed to count how many they had eaten at least once in their lives. The game's creators claimed that the average person had tried no more than twenty. One can imagine the crew of the Corps of Discovery looking at this list and snorting.

Haggis? Please! Talk to me when you've eaten grizzly bear.

As the list of meats given above suggests, the Lewis and Clark expedition was heavily carnivorous. Meat was the most concentrated source of energy available to the men, who required a huge number of calories every day to support hours of rowing, marching, hunting, and other activities. It is estimated that each member of the party burned roughly five thousand calories a day. About sixty percent of that requirement was supplied by the estimated six pounds of meat and/or fish that each man consumed in a typical day on the move.

No other food type could have fueled the men as well as flesh did, given their circumstances. There had been no agricultural revolution in the Native American nations. They were still principally hunter-gatherers. Not one field of cultivated wheat did the Corps of Discovery pass as it rowed up the Missouri River. Lewis and Clark and their men therefore became hunter-gatherers too as they traveled through the untamed territories of the "Indians." The white men were able to trade for corn at their winter base at Fort Mandan, but the majority of the cereal grain they consumed during their journey was the flour and hardtack they brought with them.

Lewis and Clark had nothing against fruits and vegetables—they reported in their journals that they quite enjoyed some of the plant foods, familiar and novel, that they tasted during their trek—but it just didn't make practical sense for the men to go out of their way to acquire them. The contribution of veggies to the travelers' micronutrient needs got a boost when the Native American woman Sacagawea joined their mission. Unlike the white men, she knew where to look for the starchy roots that were carbohydrate staples for her people. She also knew which edible-seeming plants were in fact poisonous. Wild licorice, currants, and breadroot were among the plant foods that became supplements to the men's meat-centered diet thanks to the expert scavenging efforts of their squaw companion.

The party worked their way through a sequence of distinct diets during their journey. What they ate changed by location and season and was influenced also by whether they were moving or camped and whether they were alone or in contact with native tribes. Between the late spring and early fall on the high plains, ripe fruits of many kinds were enjoyed as snacks and desserts. During the winter of 1804–1805 the men survived largely on corn acquired through trade with the Mandan Indians in the territory that later became North Dakota. At the center of each sequential diet was some savior staple, such as corn, that supplied most of their calories and without which they would have been screwed.

During brief periods of want the Corps of Discovery was more or less vegetarian, while at other times it was almost wholly carnivorous. The winter weather on the northern plains was so brutal in January 1805 that hunting was almost impossible and the travelers thus became unwilling herbivores. The following winter, which the expedition spent encamped on the Pacific Coast, the men survived almost entirely on elk meat. They built a smoke house and ate elk jerky for breakfast, lunch, and dinner day after day. The monotony nearly drove them crazy. It is telling that humans can be driven to the brink of madness by having only one thing to eat.

The Corps of Discovery Expedition was an exercise in adaptation, and the ability of its participants to adapt dietetically was the salient factor in the mission's success. Perhaps the most interesting instance of dietary adaptation in the two-year expedition was the camas root episode. The camas root was a staple of the Nez Perce, a native tribe that Lewis and Clark first encountered after a miserable crossing of the Rockies during which the travelers nearly starved. The Nez Perce fed the roots in various forms to the famished men and the men gobbled them up. Soon thereafter, they developed terrible stomach pains that left them incapacitated for days. The unfamiliar food contained indigestible fibers that produced gaseous compounds upon interaction with the men's digestive systems. But the stomachs of the Nez Perce seemed to have adapted somehow, for they swallowed the roots without complaint.

Months later, the expedition encountered the Nez Perce again as the white men made their way back east, and again they were fed camas roots. This time, however, the men were able to digest them without discomfort. Their stomachs had adapted too. New research suggests what probably happened was that the composition of the bacteria in the men's digestive tracts changed in response to their first exposure to camas roots. Scientists are discovering that the extreme responsiveness of gut flora to changes in diet are a major contributor to humans' dietary adaptability.

Remarkably, few alimentary misadventures worse than the camas root episode befell the party despite the extreme adventurousness of their eating. There were cases of scurvy and dysentery and such along the way, but when the men arrived in St. Louis in September 1806, almost two and a half years after they had set out, they were in fine fettle. One of the greatest physical achievements in human history was fueled by the broadest possible range of diets.

The Journey of Man

The expedition of Lewis and Clark was a sort of microcosmic echo of a previous expedition undertaken by the whole human race—the so-called Journey of Man. If the greater journey hadn't happened first, the smaller expedition could not have happened later.

I described the origin of the Journey of Man in Chapter 1. It began in the heart of Africa more than six million years ago. Central Africa before that time featured a balance of lush rainforests and arid grasslands. Then came a period of climatic drying that caused the grasslands to intrude upon forested territory and may have brought some hungry apes tentatively out of the trees to seek sustenance on the ground. A handful of these apes were good enough at scavenging carcasses and digging up roots to make a real go of it. From that point forward, selective survival produced generations that were increasingly well adapted to life on the floor. Originally designed to live on fruit and insects, these apes retained their ability to eat those foods while evolving to become hunters (upright posture, opposable thumbs) and meat eaters (shorter digestive tracts, stronger jaws) as well.

Anatomically modern humans came out the far end of this evolutionary process roughly 200,000 years ago. Perhaps only a few thousand members of our species existed at that time and all of them were in eastern and/or southern Africa. Every human being alive today is a direct descendent of a single woman who lived in Africa between 100,000 and 150,000 years ago. We know this because there is a particular mutation in the mitochondrial DNA of every human—which is passed down through the mother—that, like all such mutations, must have originated with a single person, and since these types of mutations tend to accumulate in the species at a steady rate, it is possible to roughly fix each one's date of origin. The fact that all of us descended from a single woman living between 100,000 and 150,000 years ago does not mean that this woman was the only woman on earth at the time. It just means that, of the hundreds or maybe thousands of women living then, only her descendents survive today.

There is a similar marker in the DNA of the Y chromosome, which is passed down from fathers to sons. This particular mutation exists in every male human living today, indicating that every human of either gender living today is a direct descendent of the man in whom this mutation first appeared. It is estimated that this man lived between 120,000 and 160,000 years ago in Africa. Although this man and the one woman from whom all living humans are descended were roughly contemporaneous, it is extremely unlikely that they knew each other, in the biblical sense or otherwise. We know this "genetic Adam" lived and died in Africa because the oldest human fossil remains outside of Africa are much younger. Human migration out of Africa appears to have begun in earnest about 60,000 years ago. Only 10,000 years later—the blink of an eye on the evolutionary time scale—humans were living as far away as Australia. And by 8,000 B.C.E. humans had reached every corner of the globe with the exception of Antarctica.

Scientists can't say with certainty why the Journey of Man happened when it did, but they have a pretty good idea. Archeological evidence indicates that at least three major changes occurred around the time the journey began: people began making more sophisticated tools, art was invented, and humans became more skillful hunters who were capable of killing a greater diversity of prey in larger numbers. Together these changes are referred to as the Great Leap Forward. It is widely believed that this leap was made possible by the development of mature language skills, which in turn were made possible by sudden growth in the human brain's short-term memory capacity. This cerebral expansion occurred long after a more drastic expansion of the brain that followed the advent of cooking, as I will describe in the next chapter, and was probably fueled by incremental improvements in cooking methods.

Grazing animals tend to migrate in search of the best pastures as seasons change (in the short term) and as climatic conditions shift (in the long term). With their newly acquired tools and abilities, humans probably began to migrate out of Africa in pursuit of their favorite prey. Interestingly, it appears that coastal-dwelling humans who lived primarily off foods from the sea got the earliest start and made the quickest progress. This makes sense if you consider that one of the main barriers to human migration would have been geographical features and environmental conditions that humans of the time were not well adapted to. Both geography and environmental conditions change more drastically inland than they do along the coast. The overall migration patterns of early humans reflect a clear desire to minimize the need to adapt, and migration along the coast was the obvious path of least resistance in this regard.

Even so, a tremendous amount of adaptation was required as our ancestors moved up the east coast of Africa and along the southern coast of Asia toward the islands that comprise Australasia, which can be reached only by boat. Humans were able to make the adaptations necessary to continue their rapid march (and float) across the planet because of the inherent adaptability they had acquired in Africa. Try as they might to keep eating what was most familiar, our migrating ancestors would have been halted altogether if they had been unwilling or unable to eat a great variety of foods, among them many novel foods. Far from being halted altogether, they fairly raced to the far ends of the earth.

The biologist Gary Paul Nabhan has spent much of his career studying the diversity of ancient human diets. "Inevitably," he has concluded, "there must have been significant turnovers in the composition of ancestral diets as our progenitors moved through space as well as through time. . . . [V]ery few foodstuffs could have been shared by ancestral peoples who contemporaneously ranged from Africa to what is now the East Indies."

Nabhan's favorite case in point is the island of Java and its neighboring islands, which migrating humans would have reached not long before their discovery of Australia. Nabhan has noted that some of the islands in this area, including Bali, are moist and tropical, while others, such as Lombok, just a few miles away, are arid. The flora and fauna in these two types of environment are starkly different. The first humans to sail from one island to the other, which would have taken no more than a few hours, would have been required to immediately assume a wholly new diet. Because they were human, it wasn't a problem.

But the adaptations required of these early island hoppers were nothing compared to those demanded of the intrepid bands of humans who broke off and ventured north—way north—instead of staying close to shore. No group went farther in that direction than did the Chukchi, who settled in northern Siberia, inside the Arctic Circle, approximately 20,000 years ago. Nighttime winter temperatures in the area approach –100 degrees Fahrenheit. The ground is frosted over ten months of every year. That leaves two months for the Chukchi to get all of their vegetable nutrition for the year: berries, wild sorrel, roseroot, and mushrooms (which are technically a fungus). Little else grows in the Chukchi territory except lichen, and the Chukchi don't eat that. But reindeer eat it, and the Chukchi eat the reindeer, prizing their lichen-packed intestines. During the winter, their only source of nourishment is fish and sea mammals such as walrus.

About 10,000 years before humans reached northern Siberia from Southeast Asia by land, the cousins of these people reached Papua New Guinea from the same point of origin by sea. They encountered an island that offered little in the way of animal foods, lacking large mammals and fish, but which was abundant in plant foods, with 650 edible species to choose from. By necessity these settlers became mostly vegetarian. This was no more a problem for the Papua New Guineans than becoming mostly carnivorous would later be for their cousins the Chukchi, with whom they shared common forebears in Southeast Asia.

Not long after humans penetrated into northern Siberia, an ice age took hold, soaking up much of the world's water and lowering the sea level. A land bridge was created at the Bering Strait, connecting Siberia to what is now known as Alaska. Naturally, humans crossed it and then quickly spread across North, Central, and South America, eventually becoming Aztecs, Sioux, and other New World peoples. Many strange foods were encountered, and as always the people who encountered them adapted their diets to encompass them.

For example, corn (or maize) was encountered in Central America. The Mayans figured out how to cook it, and it became a key staple that later spread by trade throughout the Americas. When it reached the Northern Plains, the Mandan developed an innovative method of storing excess corn from summer harvests in large, buried caches for use during the long, cold winter. In the winter of 1804–1805, cached corn from the latest harvest was shared with a group of thirty-three white men who arrived at that point on earth by way of their own lines of descent and having taken precisely the opposite route to that of their cousins the Mandans, fellow direct descendants of a single woman and (separately) a single man who lived in Africa tens of thousands of years earlier. The dietary stories of the two peoples were as disparate as their travel routes, but the corn nourished all of them equally.

From Diet to Cuisines
The foods on the list of 100 Foods to Eat Before You Die represent cuisines from all over the world. Borscht comes from Eastern

Europe, chile relleno comes from Mexico, pho comes from Vietnam, oxtail soup comes from England, and so forth. The viability of the 100 Foods to Eat Before You Die game depends on a fairly recent phenomenon: the availability of most of the world's cultural cuisines in places other than the places they come from. I've eaten baba ghanoush, for example, but I've never eaten it in the Levant.

As any American who has dined at an Ethiopian restaurant knows, and as any Frenchman who has visited Vietnam can attest, the world's various traditional cultural cuisines are quite different from one another. The characteristic diets of the world's peoples began to take shape in the Neolithic Age. Not long after humans reached the four corners of the earth, the development of agriculture caused populations to settle down where they were and form complex societies. The interaction of locally available foods, cultural factors, and advancing methods of food production gave birth to cuisines that were as different from those of other peoples as they were from the diets of all pre-Neolithic humans.

Modern analysis of traditional cuisines has revealed that they differ nutritionally as much as they do in their ingredients and flavors. Let's look at a few examples.

In a master's degree thesis submitted to the University of Montana, Margit Elisabeth Groessler analyzed the traditional diet of the Saalish, Kootenai, and Pend d'Oreille Indians of northwest Montana prior to 1806, the very year the Lewis and Clark expedition came to an end. According to Groessler, meat and fish accounted for approximately 70 percent of the calories in the diet of these people. They hunted bison, elk, deer, moose, and fowl and fished for salmon. Their plant staples changed by season. In the early spring, potatoes, wild celery, wild carrots, watercress, and bitterroot were predominant. In the late spring and early summer, there was a shift toward camas root, service berries, chokecherries, gooseberries, boysenberries, wild strawberries, and wild raspberries. In the late summer, foamberries and huckleberries were plentiful.

Because the traditional diet of the Saalish, Kootenai, and Pend d'Oreille Indians had vanished by the time Groessler conducted her nutritional analysis, she had to base it on the best possible reconstruction she could create. She had a fairly exhaustive list of the foods these tribes had eaten, and she was confident in the 70 percent meat and fish figure, so the data she came up with are probably accurate. Groessler calculated that the traditional diet of the natives of northwestern Montana was roughly 50 percent protein, 30 percent carbohydrate, and 20 percent fat. This is a very high-protein diet. Protein accounts for only 18 percent of calories in the typical American diet today.

Contrast this to the traditional diet of the inhabitants of Crete, which is the model for what has become known as the Mediterranean diet. It was first analyzed by the American epidemiologist Leland Allbaugh in 1948. Crete was not an island of plenty at that time, and few Cretans could afford to eat much meat. Allbaugh's analysis revealed that 61 percent of the calories in the Cretan diet came from fruits, vegetables, greens, nuts, and roots. Most of the remaining calories came from olive oil, which was eaten with just about everything. Allbaugh reported that Cretans consumed nearly four tablespoons of olive oil per day. Animal foods such as fish, lamb, rabbit, and snails accounted for only 10 percent of their calories.

In terms of macronutrients, the traditional Cretan diet is best described as a high-fat diet. Fat accounted for 40 percent of daily calories, carbohydrate for 45 percent, and protein for the remaining 15 percent. Although fat is widely considered to be unhealthy, Cretans at the time of Allbaugh's study had the lowest incidence of heart disease anywhere on earth.

The macronutrient breakdown of the traditional Hawaiian diet is very different from those of both the Cretan diet and the diet of the Native Americans of northwestern Montana. Hawaii was one of the last places on earth to be inhabited by humans, and it's no mystery why: the Hawaiian Islands are 2,000 miles from the nearest continental land mass. The first settlers are believed to have arrived there from Polynesia between 4,000 and 2,500 years ago. Hawaii could not have been their intended destination because those first settlers could not have known it existed, but they were certainly prepared for a long journey. Several staples of the traditional Hawaiian diet—including pork and taro root—are not native to the island. The first settlers must have carried these foods to sustain themselves through weeks or months at sea and then introduced them to the island when they landed.

Most of the foods of the traditional Hawaiian diet, including seaweed, fish, and coconuts, are indigenous to the islands. So the diet that the Polynesian adventurers adopted upon settling there would have been necessarily very different from their diet back home. Like native Hawaiian civilization as a whole, the traditional Hawaiian diet was all but wiped out by the European takeover that began with the arrival of Captain Cook in 1778. In the 1990s Hawaiian physicians Terry Shintani and Sheila Beckham reconstructed the traditional Hawaiian diet in an effort to combat the epidemic of obesity that had followed the natives' transition to a modern Western diet. Leaning on taro, sweet potato, fern shoots, seaweed, native fruits, fish, and fowl, this diet is undoubtedly very close to that which sustained Native Hawaiians until the twentieth century. It is a very high-carbohydrate diet, with a macronutrient breakdown of 78 percent carbohydrate, 15 percent protein, and 7 percent fat.

All of the available evidence suggests that each of the three cultural diets I've just described nourished more than adequately the people who traditionally ate it. As I mentioned, the high-fat diet of the people of Crete rewarded them with the lowest rate of heart disease in the world as of the mid-twentieth century.

While the health of many Native American peoples has been destroyed by an abrupt switch to the modern Western diet, the greatest health complaints of the natives of northwest Montana in the past were related to hunger during times of scarcity when they were unable to sustain the high-protein diet that normally kept them in the pink.

The healthfulness of the traditional Hawaiian diet for Native Hawaiians is backed by research. In 1991 Terry Shintani and Sheila Beckham placed twenty Native Hawaiians with multiple cardiovascular disease risk factors on a traditional Hawaiian diet for twenty-one days. The subjects were allowed to eat as much as they wanted, but they were only allowed to eat foods that were available on the islands before contact with Europeans. In just three weeks the Native Hawaiians lost an average of seventeen pounds and experienced significant reductions in total cholesterol and blood pressure.

Clearly the traditional Hawaiian diet was good for Native Hawaiians, the traditional Cretan diet was good for the aboriginal inhabitants of that island, and the traditional diet of the Native Americans of northwestern Montana was good for them. But could a Native Hawaiian be just as healthy on the traditional Saalish or Cretan diet? Could a Cretan or Kootenai remain as robust on the Native Hawaiian diet? The three diets we've looked at ranged from 30 to 78 percent carbohydrate, 7 to 40 percent fat, and 15 to 50 percent protein. So here's the real question: Could a human being of *any* ancestry be equally healthy on a diet of natural foods whose macronutrient breakdown fell anywhere within these broad ranges?

There is no reason to believe otherwise. True, geneticists have found clear evidence of ethnic adaptation to specific traditional diets. For example, genes that protect against excessive intoxication and alcoholism are far more widespread in peoples whose traditional diet included alcoholic beverages than they are in Native

American populations, which consumed little or no alcohol. So it would be a bridge too far to suggest that any person on earth could thrive on any traditional diet. But factors such as alcohol sensitivity are really rather marginal. By and large, thanks to our special history, human beings can eat in any number of different ways and be equally healthy.

While researching his book *Why Some Like It Hot: Food, Genes, and Cultural Diversity*, Gary Paul Nabhan, whom I mentioned earlier, made a visit to Crete with his wife. For duty and for pleasure the couple ate like Cretans, not excluding their daily allotment of several tablespoons of olive oil. After a few days both of them were suffering from upset stomachs and had to back off the olive oil for a while. Later, Nabhan learned from Antonis Kafatos, a nutrition researcher at the University of Crete, that it takes three or four weeks for outsiders to adapt to such high levels of olive oil consumption. In one study Kafatos had found that Cretans were initially able to clear excess lipids from their blood much faster after consuming olive oil than were British subjects placed on a Cretan diet. But after a few weeks this discrepancy had disappeared. The Brits had adapted to the Cretan diet, much as Lewis and Clark had adapted to camas roots two centuries earlier.

Lots of studies have looked at the effects of Mediterranean diets, like the traditional Cretan way of eating, on various health parameters in other ethnic populations. Most of the participants in these studies have switched to the Mediterranean diet not from other traditional cultural diets but rather from modern diets packed with processed foods. One such study, known as the northern Manhattan study, involved a subject pool that was 55 percent Hispanic, 21 percent white, and 24 percent black. The researchers conducting the study discovered that, over a nine-year period, the subjects who stuck to the Mediterranean diet most faithfully had the lowest risk of stroke and heart attack. So apparently you don't have to be a Cretan to benefit from eating like one.

The Myth of One True Way

The first principle of the healthy-diet cults is the idea that there is a single right way to eat for optimal health. The fact of the matter is that the evolutionary history of our species has left us with the ability to adapt to a multiplicity of diets. This ability was exploited and consummated in the Journey of Man, whereby humanity dispersed from Africa to populate the entire earth between 60,000 and 5,000 years ago. Lewis and Clark later took the adaptability of the human diet for granted in planning and executing their expedition across North America. And in our own time, the creators of the Facebook game 100 Foods to Eat Before You Die would never have come up with the idea if the same understanding did not exist somewhere deep within each of us.

By no means am I suggesting that human beings can eat whatever they please without suffering negative health consequences, especially in a food environment such as ours today that is marked by a superabundance of cheap, tasty, high-calorie processed goodies. Nutrition science has proven with great redundancy that eating for optimal health is not an "anything goes" proposition. You can see this for yourself by peeking inside your local McDonald's during the noon rush and observing the shapes and sizes of the people eating there. The historical examples we have examined in this chapter are not meant to contradict such glaring evidence from the laboratory and the nearest McDonald's.

What our history does show us is that, despite the messages we receive from the many contending preachers of the One True Way, there are numerous dietary pathways to optimal health. Ironically, it is this very breadth of options that makes it possible for the various healthy-diet cults to produce good results that support the illusion of their superiority.

3

Homo Coquus

Bernie Freeman lives by the motto "Go hard or go home." His penchant for extremes is expressed in all facets of his life, including his health habits. Throughout his adult years, Bernie has pinballed between phases of Jack LaLanne-like dedication to fitness and periods of Homer Simpsonesque gluttony. Not so long ago, Bernie was living on cheeseburgers and beer. Today he is a raw vegan.

Like all of us, Bernie owes his disposition partly to heredity and partly to upbringing—nature and nurture. He grew up in eastern Washington State with two brothers, neither of whom shared his obsessive-compulsive tendencies. For better or worse, nature had lit a fire inside Bernie that it had not in his siblings. The father of the three boys was a cop, a real man's man, and a stern paterfamilias. Throughout his childhood Bernie looked up to his dad and sought to emulate him and make him proud. Over time, this drive to win respect became generalized, something Bernie directed at everyone whose good opinion mattered to him.

In high school Bernie played football and golf, excelling in both sports, golf especially. He was offered a scholarship to play in college, but after one year he happened to see a pack of military helicopters flying in formation over a fairway he was standing on and instantly decided to drop out of college, join the Army, and fly helicopters.

Imperfect eyesight prevented Bernie from becoming a pilot, so he became a paratrooper instead. By the time he completed jump school, he had developed an insatiable need to continuously push the envelope of his toughness. A little bit of cheating death was fine, but more was always better. This hunger led Bernie almost inevitably to Ranger School, a sixty-one-day elite Army leadership training program that presses candidates to the brink of physical collapse and mental implosion. More than half of every Ranger class fails to complete the program, and Bernie's class was no exception. But he made it through.

Some of Bernie's Special Forces buddies were avid cyclists. He started to ride with them and discovered he had a gift for going long. Endurance sports suddenly presented themselves to him as a terrific new way to explore his toughness. Bernie decided to become a triathlete and got himself stationed in Hawaii, where he could train hard year-round. His first race was an Ironman-distance event on Oahu, which he won. The Army took notice and reassigned Bernie to a sinecure—a job in name only that left him free to train all day long, which he dutifully did. Between Friday and Sunday of each week he completed the equivalent of a full Ironman triathlon—2.4 miles of swimming, 112 miles of cycling, and 26.2 miles of running. The rest of the week was marginally tamer, spreading a second Ironman's worth of training across four days. The same fanaticism that had helped Bernie become an Army Ranger he now poured into his training.

The king of triathlon in the 1980s was Dave Scott, six-time winner of the Ironman World Championship. Scott was not only a legendary trainaholic but also a fanatically clean eater who weighed his food and famously rinsed his cottage cheese to reduce its fat content. Bernie bought and read Scott's book and began to emulate his diet. He counted every single calorie he swallowed to ensure that he maintained a consistent macronutrient breakdown of 60 percent carbohydrate, 20 percent fat, and 20 percent protein. He went years without eating cheese because it messed up the ratio.

After finishing fourteenth at Ironman Canada, Bernie decided that this was the life for him. He registered for the Army Master Fitness Trainer Course and graduated at the top of his class, correctly answering 497 out of 500 questions in the final exam. Soon afterward he landed a marketing job with a startup sports nutrition company called PowerBar.

Bernie threw himself into his work for PowerBar as completely as he had previously thrown himself into golf, the Army, and triathlon. He developed an innovative field marketing program that helped the company grow from a seat-of-the-pants regional operation into a global juggernaut with tens of millions of dollars in annual revenues. But along the way he ran into an irony that is familiar to men and women who are led into the business of sport by a personal passion for sport: he no longer had time to train.

The slide was subtle at first. Bernie held on to the semblance of an athlete's physique by continuing to eat like Dave Scott even though he barely ever worked out anymore. But his occasional cheeseburger "cheat" meals became increasingly frequent until they were no longer exceptions but the rule. By the time Bernie left PowerBar to start his own sports marketing business, the ex-Ranger who had effectively been doing two Ironmans a week was overweight and out of shape.

There followed several short-lived comeback attempts. Suddenly fed up with himself, Bernie would abruptly stop eating cheeseburgers and drinking beer and dust off his bike. During one of these brief comebacks, Bernie went for a ride with a mixed-gender group of unspectacular athletes and suffered the humiliation of getting dropped on a hill climb. Remembering the days when he could hammer out a forty-kilometer time trial in fifty-six minutes, he almost cried.

Years passed. Before he knew it Bernie was staring ahead at his fiftieth birthday. He was at least fifty pounds overweight. Enough was enough. He went back on the Dave Scott diet, bought a new bike, and embarked upon his most earnest comeback attempt yet. The weight fell off in globs. He was turning back the clock. This time it was different—he was going to take it all the way!

That feeling lasted about six weeks. He just couldn't sustain it. The spark somehow wasn't there like it used to be. As his motivation to continue his comeback flagged, Bernie began to suspect that he had lost something in all those years of jumping out of airplanes and racing marathons and triathlons. A little more time passed and he felt certain of it.

Once again, Bernie reacquainted himself with cheeseburgers and beer and quickly regained the weight he'd lost. Then a thought occurred to him—an idea so simple, he almost couldn't believe it hadn't occurred to him sooner.

Why not try something different?

Instead of struggling to go backward and reclaim what he had lost, perhaps he could go forward along a new path toward better health!

But which path? There was only one way to find it: YouTube. Bernie logged onto his favorite website for research, punched in all kinds of diet- and health-related search terms, and watched scores of videos proclaiming dozens of solutions, mostly dietary. The sheer variety of paths toward better health available to him was briefly paralyzing, but Bernie had faith in his intuitions, and these led him to a solution that felt surprisingly right: raw food.

On the surface it seemed a bizarre choice. Most of the raw-food advocates Bernie encountered on YouTube were tree-hugging hippie types, whereas Bernie's hero was Ronald Reagan. Beyond that, raw-foodism was a hardcore subspecies of vegetarianism, and Bernie had never been remotely attracted to a life without meat. But the raw diet was also very much an all-or-nothing proposition, and Bernie was attracted to that. He had thrived on the rigid structure imposed by the Army and the athletic lifestyle, and this raw-food diet offered something similar. There was also something about the concept of superfoods, which raw-foodists were always carrying on about, that appealed to Bernie. But the strongest attraction of the raw diet for Bernie was the simple fact that it required no cooking.

In all his years on the Dave Scott diet and beyond, Bernie had never learned to cook anything more complicated than a pot of spaghetti. He hated cooking. What little laziness there was in him was concentrated in the culinary dimension of his life. Bernie would almost rather starve than follow a recipe. The raw diet was a diet that forbade cooking. So in a weird way it was a perfect match for a microwave bachelor like Bernie.

Eating Clean

One of the raw-food advocates Bernie discovered on YouTube was Dan McDonald, a.k.a. Dan the Man, a.k.a. the Life Regenerator. Dan had been a raw-foodist for about a dozen years and had been a professional raw-food crusader for almost as long when Bernie found him. His prolific output of video sermons on the virtues of raw food, all of them featuring Dan's winsomely mellow evangelism, had attracted legions of followers.

In one of the videos available on his YouTube channel (which was closing in on fourteen million views when Bernie first watched it), Dan appeared in a white T-shirt on which his personal and professional motto was imprinted in black lettering:

> alkalize.
> detoxify.
> regenerate.

It struck Bernie that Dan could have played Jesus in a Hollywood movie. He had long straight hair, a neatly trimmed beard, and a handsomely carved face. He was quite thin—almost undernourished-looking, actually, but perhaps this was only because (as Dan explained at the beginning of the video) he was in the middle of a "water fast" when he filmed this particular piece.

The twenty-two-minute monologue Dan delivered was extemporaneous and somewhat rambling (a fault he apologized for more than once), very loosely structured as a point-by-point dissertation on the three words of his motto. Dan looked down at his T-shirt frequently to keep himself on track, as a completely different sort of presenter might look at a PowerPoint slide.

"People think you need all this protein," he said, "but I'll tell you what: 80 percent of the people with diseases that I work with have eaten *too much* protein and it's rotting and it's fermenting and it's rancidifying in their body, creating odors under their arms, clogging up the vision, clogging up the lymphatic system, occluding the heart, rotting and fermenting in all the cracks and corners and crevices in the body. You want to be clean, my friend. You want to be *clean*."

As a subspecies of vegetarianism, raw-foodism is animated by the belief that eating animal foods is unhealthy and is not something that our species was "meant" to do. Raw-food advocates often point out that our species' closest animal relative, the bonobo, with which we share a 98 percent genetic overlap, is an

herbivore. They also like to observe that the human body is anatomically and physiologically more like those of herbivores than
of carnivores in the animal kingdom. Carnivores have sharp front
teeth to tear flesh; humans do not. Our intestinal tract, they note,
is structurally more similar to a lamb's than a lion's. Our stomach
acids, too, are poorly suited to the digestion of meat compared
to those produced by the stomachs of 100 percent meat-eaters.

On all of these points, raw-foodists and non-raw vegetarians
agree. Where the two cults part ways is on the matter of cooking.
Raw-foodists believe that cooked food of any kind is every bit as
unnatural and unhealthy as meat. This idea was first proposed
more than a century ago by Maximilian Bircher-Benner, a Swiss
medical doctor and spiritual father of the raw-food movement. Born
in 1867, Bircher-Benner was strongly influenced as a young man by
the German *Lebensreform* movement, a back-to-nature social wave
that sought to reverse the unhealthy effects of mankind's modern
divorce from nature. A diverse coalition, *Lebensreform* encompassed
holistic medicine, nudism, free love, alternative spirituality,
hiking, and Bircher-Benner's main interest: diet.

In 1891 Bircher-Benner received a medical degree from the
University of Zurich. Over the next few years he became increasingly interested in vegetarian diets. But his own experimentation
with meatless eating taught him that it did not go far enough. He
decided that a vegetarian diet based on raw foods was necessary
for optimal health. After all, other animals ate only raw foods,
and Charles Darwin had shown that humans shared a common
origin with those animals. So if we *really* wanted to go back to
nature in our eating habits, we had to go raw.

In 1904 Bircher-Benner opened a sanatorium in the Swiss Alps
and named it Lebendinge Kraft, or "Life Force." Patients there
were required to accept a mostly raw vegetarian diet whose chief
staple was a stew that combined shredded apples, oat flakes, cream,
honey, chopped nuts, and lemon juice. This dish became known

(and is still known today) as Bircher muesli. The term "Life Force" had a special meaning in the Lebensreform culture. It referred to solar energy, which was thought to exist in greater concentration in plant foods than in meat. Bircher-Benner, as was his wont, went further, preaching that solar energy was diminished not only by the incorporation of plants into meat but also by cooking. Raw plant foods were therefore healthier than cooked foods of any kind.

There was, of course, no evidence that the life force that Bircher-Benner deemed all-important actually existed. His peers in the mainstream medical establishment dismissed the life-force concept as unscientific and branded Bircher-Benner a quack. But it hardly mattered. The Life Force Sanatorium thrived until Bircher-Benner's (rather early) death in 1939, and kept going for some time even after his passing.

By that time, raw-foodism had made the inevitable leap across the Atlantic to the United States, where it was popularized by the likes of Ann Wigmore, who is credited with coining the term "living foods." Although the raw-food movement has experienced a second growth spurt in recent years, it remains very small, largely because it is incredibly difficult to sustain a 100 percent raw diet. Even Dan the Man has confessed to falling a couple of points short of perfection.

"Once in a while I will do things that aren't the best, and I regret it," he ruefully told the camera in his water-fast video.

The popularity of raw-foodism is constrained not only by its sheer difficulty but also by its continued lack of scientific endorsement. As Bernie Freeman discovered in his YouTube research, formally trained nutrition scientists do not advocate raw-foodism, and the typical raw-food advocate is as about as likely to have a mainstream nutrition credential as is the typical fast-food restaurant manager. None of the authors of the several popular books on raw-foodism holds even a dietetics certification, let alone a doctoral degree in nutrition. Dan the Man himself has admitted to wishing he "had more science."

Most raw-food advocates really couldn't care less about science and blithely continue to talk about life-force energy. But some have bent to the pressures of the times and tried to make scientific-sounding arguments in favor of raw food. One such argument states that cooking destroys the natural enzymes that aid digestion and nutrient uptake when food is eaten raw. But in fact, the enzymes in foods are rendered biologically inert by digestion, whether the foods that contain them are eaten cooked or raw. They don't do anything once absorbed into the human body.

A second argument contends that cooking destroys vital nutrients in foods. However, real science suggests that something close to the opposite is true. For example, a 2012 study conducted by researchers at the University of Wisconsin found that cooking increased the bioavailability of vitamin A in bananas. Cooking also greatly increases the amount of energy that the body is able to extract from foods. (I'll return to this point a bit later.)

Yet another pro-raw argument says that cooking introduces toxic compounds to foods. Cooking is indeed known to create advanced glycation end-products (or AGEs), which have been implicated in the development of inflammatory conditions and gestational diabetes. Other toxic chemicals created by cooking include trans fats, heterocyclic amines, acrylamide, and nitrosamines. Raw-foodists make much of these toxins. Dan the Man says we're "killing ourselves" when we eat cooked food. He has a point with respect to frying. Consumption of fried foods really needs to be kept to a minimum if maximum health is to be preserved. But it is not necessary to avoid cooked foods generally to keep the intake of the most harmful cooking-related toxins within safe limits. French fries contain more than 200 times the amount of AGEs that are in a bowl of oatmeal, although both are cooked. Experts agree that a diet which includes few fried foods and an otherwise normal mix of cooked and raw foods will not shorten life by the sort of poisoning that raw-foodists fear.

In addition to pointing out the mostly imaginary dangers of cooked foods, raw-foodists cite a long list of health benefits associated with their way of eating. These include weight loss; reduced risk of diabetes, cancer, and heart disease; better digestion; lower cholesterol; improved skin appearance; and more positive mood states. There's very little scientific research to support most of these claims. One thing is certain, though: raw-foodists are generally very pleased with the results of their diet. A 2006 survey of nearly 900 raw-foodists found that the elimination of cooked foods from the diet was commonly perceived to have resulted in fat loss, improved digestion and regularity, increased sleep quality, higher energy levels, and improved mood state and mental health.

Anecdotally, raw-foodists almost universally report an additional benefit that is all but impossible to quantify: a feeling of energy, lightness, vitality, and clarity that is often observable to others as a visible radiance.

"I want you to feel that energy of life that I feel flowing through me right now," said Dan the Man in his water-fast video. "I want to pass it to you."

Bernie could see that energy of life flowing through the man. Gaunt though he was, the Life Regenerator was undeniably radiant.

Hungry but Happy

After deciding to "go raw," Bernie spent a good two weeks planning and preparing for his new lifestyle. First he cleaned out his kitchen. He ransacked his pantry, emptying it of foods that did not make the cut as defined by his new eating rules. Boxes, cans, and cartons of perfectly good, non-raw food—some of them not yet opened—went straight into a big black Hefty bag. Nothing was spared. Bernie then threw open the doors of his refrigerator and freezer and repeated the exercise. A fundamentally frugal man who ordinarily winced at waste, Bernie took pleasure in this deliberate purging. The real waste, he understood, had been committed when the food was purchased; getting rid of it now added nothing to the original sin.

Kitchen emptied, Bernie set out on a big grocery-shopping expedition. Over the next couple of days he restocked his refrigerator with fresh, raw produce. A few new items—nuts, seeds, and some healthy oils—were added to the pantry, but the cupboards remained relatively bare, as most raw eaters' cupboards are. Bernie also bought two small appliances that no raw-foodist's kitchen is complete without: a blender and a juicer.

The first several days of Bernie's new diet were a process of trial and error. Some ideas didn't work out. Kale tasted nasty in the smoothies that were the foundation of Bernie's new diet, so he stopped buying it and settled on spinach as his go-to green for liquefaction. Within a week Bernie had worked out a daily regimen that, while defying raw-food orthodoxy in a few ways, suited him.

Each morning upon waking, Bernie squeezed some fresh lemon into a big glass of filtered water and guzzled it. No more coffee. Dan the Man and many other raw-foodists are big on hydrating as a vehicle for detoxification and as a way to deal with the gnawing hunger that attends the raw way of life. Bernie fell into a routine of drinking a gallon of cold green tea (a superfood) each day in addition to his early-morning glass of water with lemon.

Breakfast was a smoothie that combined so many superfoods that it took more than ten minutes to prepare despite being uncooked. The recipe varied depending on what was available in the refrigerator. A typical concoction contained fresh apple juice, a banana, fresh berries, spinach, powdered maca, cacao, goji berries, chia seeds, chlorophyll, spirulina, apple vinegar, and flax oil. Lunch was a giant salad with more spinach, tomatoes, avocado, and garbanzo beans dressed (heretically) with Boathouse Farms Yogurt Dressing. Dinner was another salad.

These meals were supplemented with a steady intake of cold green tea and fresh fruit snacks. Bernie found himself putting things in his mouth pretty much all day long on his new diet. If he stopped eating for longer than an hour, hunger pangs consumed his attention.

Bernie was fortunate to work at home, his computer twenty feet away from the fridge. But even with ready access to all the fresh raw fruits and vegetables he could eat, Bernie still felt distractingly hungry at times, so he added another cheat to his diet: a bowl of mixed nuts and seeds with almond milk, something no raw-food purist would touch, but it kept Bernie away from far greater lapses.

The first couple of days were fairly easy. The novelty of the raw routine drew Bernie's mind away from the pleas for fresh rations emanating from his stomach. A big surge of renewed self-esteem came as an immediate reward. Then the cravings kicked in.

Just one cheeseburger won't kill me.

Good god, can I really live like this?

But Bernie stuck to the plan, and the cravings settled down. The big rewards soon followed. The first thing Bernie noticed was an improvement in the quality of his sleep. He lost consciousness as soon as his head hit the pillow at night, he slept hard, and he woke in the morning feeling utterly refreshed. As his sleep improved, so did Bernie's energy level throughout the day. The familiar mid-morning and mid-afternoon doldrums vanished, and although hardcore exercise was not a part of his plan, Bernie found it easy to become a little more active. He also experienced the improvements in clarity of thought and mental productivity that are so common among raw-foodists. And, yes, he began to feel an indescribable inner cleanness and lightness. In the mirror he noticed a marked improvement in the tone and color of his skin. There was no other word for it: he looked radiant.

It took a few weeks for the weight loss to become noticeable— Bernie had also resolved not to weigh himself—but once it had begun, it progressed rapidly. Bernie disappeared inside increasingly baggy clothes. At his next checkup, the same doctor who had previously admonished Bernie now congratulated him.

Born to Barbecue

Humans have been eating meat since before they technically existed. Paleontologists have found animal bones bearing hack marks from stone tools that date back as far as 2.5 million years. Homo sapiens goes back only 200,000 years. It was not our species but rather our ancestors the habilenes who used those tools. The brain of the habilenes, which were the first meat-eaters in our lineage, was one third larger than the brain of the australopithecines, the last herbivores, and meat was the reason. The addition of meat to the diet of our ancient hominid ancestors greatly increased their energy intake, fueling a significant increase in brain size.

It is not known exactly when our ancestors began to cook, but the date keeps moving back. A recent archeological discovery in South Africa proved that campfires existed one million years ago, or some 300,000 years earlier than previous evidence indicated. Experts including the noted primatologist Richard Wrangham believe that cooking may have started another half-million years before that, around the time habilenes were displaced by homo erectus. These scientists note that the brain of homo erectus was more than 40 percent larger than that of the habilenes. Only the advent of cooking, they say, could have provided enough energy to fuel such explosive growth in brain size, especially after meat was already well entrenched in the diet.

Support for the early-cooking theory continues to accumulate. In 2012, for example, Wrangham disclosed new evidence that more than two million years ago, our ancestors used smoke to keep bees from stinging them when gathering honey. If scientists eventually are able to confirm with certainty that we've been cooking since that far back, then the fundamental premise of the raw-food diet—that human beings are "meant" to base their diet on raw foods—is as wrong as it could possibly be. Cooking actually *made us human*. The invention of cooking improved the diet quality of our ancestors in ways that drastically increased their brain power and elevated them above other primates. The human brain (as well as other parts of the body) evolved through the medium of cooking and remains to this day deeply adapted to a diet of cooked food. The scientific name of our species is *homo sapiens*—"knowing man." Perhaps it ought to have been *homo coquus*—"cooking man."

Cooking increases the energy yield of foods by denaturing proteins, gelatinizing starches, and softening foods so that they are more easily digested. Chimpanzees spend six hours a day chewing. They have to do this to get enough energy from raw jungle foods to survive. The average adult human spends less than one hour a day eating and gets significantly more energy from a far smaller volume of food than do our primate cousins. Studies have shown that animals ranging from insects to cows grow and develop much more rapidly on a diet of cooked food. The difference between us and other animals is that we have been eating mostly cooked food for so long that our bodies have changed to take full advantage of it at the cost of becoming very much dependent on it. Our most important adaptation to cooked food is our massive brains, which never could have come to exist if not for cooking.

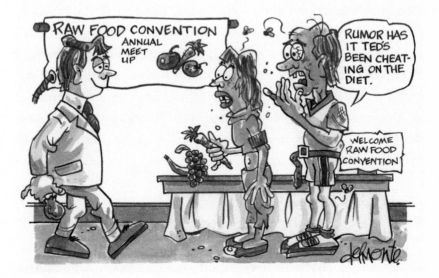

One of the reasons people today lose so much weight when they go raw is that a cooked version of any food yields so much more usable energy. A German study found that, on average, men lost 21.8 pounds and women lost 26.5 pounds after starting a raw-based diet. Those who ate the least cooked food lost the most weight. While weight loss is generally regarded as a good thing in our age of obesity, most people who go raw are not overweight and there is reason to believe that in many cases their weight loss is not entirely healthy. One third of subjects in the German study I just mentioned who ate purely raw diets were so skinny that they were medically classified as undernourished. Sixty percent of the women either ceased to menstruate or had irregular menses. They had lost so much body fat that their bodies were too weak and undernourished to procreate.

It bears mentioning that today's raw-foodists are able to take advantage of a variety of ways to increase their energy intake that our ancient ancestors would have lacked. Blending and juicing increase the energy yield of fruits and vegetables by obviating the body's need to liquefy them. The use of processed oils is perhaps more significant. The raw-foodists involved in the German study I just described got an average of 30 percent of their daily calories from uncooked oils that did not exist before "modern" times. Richard Wrangham has argued that a human being living today who went completely raw without such shortcuts might not even be able to survive. Our huge brains are just too dependent on things broiled, boiled, roasted, baked, fried, poached, and steamed. That's why our ancient ancestors, after their first taste of cooked food, never looked back.

Heretical Moderation

A few months into his new lifestyle, Bernie Freeman got sick. Frustrated, he broke his diet. It was all or nothing. Fortunately, a medication he was prescribed did its thing, and before long Bernie was ready to resume his diet, which his doctor supported.

Having learned a few lessons in the first go-around, Bernie tried some new tricks in his second attempt at raw living. To save money and reduce the frequency of his shopping excursions, he started a vegetable garden in his back yard. No green thumb, Bernie went back to YouTube to gather the required knowhow. He chose organic methods, not because he bought into the hair-on-fire alarmism of the rants of the "raw-food snobs" against non-organic foods and genetically modified organisms and Monsanto, but rather because organic gardening was simpler and cheaper than the alternative. Unlike most raw-foodists, Bernie seldom purchased organic produce. He was confident that well-washed nonorganic fruits and vegetables were just as healthy as organic ones, and they cost half as much.

Not long ago, I was living on cheeseburgers and beer, Bernie thought. *Does it really matter now whether I eat organic or nonorganic fruits and vegetables?*

Sardines were another new tool that Bernie added to his second try at raw eating. It wasn't that he craved salty tinned fish. Bernie just couldn't shake some concerns he had about the quality of plant protein, so he decided to include a little animal protein in his regimen. As a cooked animal food, sardines are doubly defiant of accepted raw-foodist practice. Bernie couldn't have cared less. While the all-or-nothing approach worked for him most of the time, in raw-foodism Bernie had finally discovered something he preferred to do in moderation, recognizing that he was less likely to go back to the "nothing" of cheeseburgers and beer if he went less than "all in" with raw food.

The Myth of Natural

All of the modern healthy-diet cults take it as given that human beings are meant to eat a certain way. Most of them agree that we are meant to eat in the most "natural" way possible. Different cults have their own definitions of "natural." Raw-foodism distinguishes itself from other natural-diet cults in labeling both meat and cooking as unnatural.

What's *really* natural for the individuals of any species is eating what the rest of the group eats. Antelope eat grass. An antelope that ate other antelope would be unnatural in his behavior. As we have seen, meat-eating and cooking are as natural for our species as are tool use and language. Humans on raw diets are therefore behaving unnaturally. They can feel it, too, as Bernie did. It has been estimated that more than 99 percent of people who go raw eventually go back, usually after discovering that the initial dam-burst of benefits, which perhaps are mainly psychological, inevitably give way to lethargy, excessive weight loss, indigestion, headaches, and ever-worsening hunger and cravings.

These facts do more than subvert the raw-foodists' belief that humans are not meant to consume meat or cooked food. They also undermine the general principle that our diet must be as natural as possible to support optimal health. Cooking is a form of food processing, after all, and cooking also made us human. Therefore, food processing in general is natural for our species. This is as true for more recent forms of food processing (from leavening and oil extraction to grain refining and hydrogenation) as it is for cooking.

To be sure, some of the newer forms of processing are problematic, particularly for persons seeking maximum health, in the modern context of food superabundance. You're not going to be very healthy if you eat french fries and drink energy drinks all day. But it is foolish to sweepingly label all forms of food processing as unhealthy. They must be considered case by case. Some forms of food processing, such as the addition of large amounts of sugar to foods, clearly make them less healthful and therefore such foods should be eaten sparingly. Other forms of food processing, such as milk culturing, enhance the nutritional value of natural foods.

The healthy-diet cults would like nothing more than for one tidy principle—be it naturalism or something else—to define what is good to eat and what is not with zero exceptions. But no such principle exists. Any specific way of eating that works for a person—whether it's Bernie Freeman's mostly-raw diet or my agnostic healthy eating—is a way of eating that *shouldn't* work according to the ideology of one or more healthy-diet cults.

4

The Caveman of Orange County

B rian MacKenzie woke up at six o'clock on a Wednesday morning in the middle of May to find his bedroom awash in sunlight. It was going to be another beautiful day. Without leaving the bed, Brian reached for his laptop and opened his email inbox, which, as always, had filled up with new messages overnight. His intention was to read only the two or three important ones, but that plan never held up, and sure enough he got sucked into going through the whole stack. As the creator and head of CrossFit Endurance, a hugely successful branch of the stupendously successful CrossFit fitness club franchise, Brian was constantly inundated from all sides with requests for bits of his attention. He had an hour to kill anyway.

At a quarter to seven, Brian shut his laptop and fed Isabella, his pit bull, and let her out to do her business. He then grabbed the key to his black Audi A6 with black rims and tinted windows and, Alice in Chains thundering, sped into downtown Laguna Beach, an upscale Orange County village hugging the Pacific Coast. Café Anastasia was just opening when Brian swaggered in, looking more like a cage fighter than a marathoner with his tattoo sleeves, granite chin, and tightly bolted 190-pound frame.

Anastasia was Brian's go-to place for a quick meal because the chefs made food to order and Brian was very particular about what he ate. This morning he ordered scrambled eggs with spinach and bacon. Anyone else might have asked for cheese on the scramble, but Brian did not, because humans have only been eating cheese for 8,000 years. Anastasia normally served home-fried potatoes with eggs, but Brian asked that his potatoes be held (actually, he didn't have to ask), because humans have only eaten potatoes for 14,000 years. And while a few slices of toast might have been a nice complement to a plate of eggs and bacon for another customer, Brian no longer ate bread, because cultivated wheat has only been a part of human diets for ten or twelve millennia.

Brian MacKenzie was on the Paleo Diet. Like the millions of other people who were following some version of the diet at the time, Brian was doing his best to eat like a caveman—or like a Paleolithic human, more accurately. Scientists place the Paleolithic period between the appearance of the first bipedal primates 2.5 million years ago and the agricultural revolution, which began sometime around 8,000 B.C.E. Since the advent of agriculture, humans by and large have eaten less and less like their Paleolithic ancestors. But in the 1970s a small number of people in the most advanced societies began to try to revive the hunter-gatherer way of eating.

The father of the movement was a gastroenterologist named Walter Voegtlin, who believed that modern humans could achieve optimal health only if they ate exclusively the same foods their Stone Age progenitors ate. For eons, he reasoned, the human genome had interacted with and adapted to these foods, which through this process had become like a set of keys to unlock our greatest vitality. In contrast, many staples of the modern diet, such as grains and dairy products, were so new to our DNA (on an evolutionary timescale) that the body scarcely new what to do with them.

The popularity of Paleolithic eating exploded after the 2002 publication of *The Paleo Diet*, whose author, Loren Cordain, worked as an exercise scientist at Colorado State University. In his book, Cordain stated in no uncertain terms that his new diet was the One True Way for everyone to eat. "With this diet, we are returning to the diet we were genetically programmed to follow," he proclaimed. "It is the closest approximation we can make, given the current scientific knowledge, to humanity's original, universal diet." The Paleo Diet gained an initial foothold with certain types of athletes before climbing on to mainstream success. It became the semi-official diet of CrossFit when a disciple of Cordain named Robb Wolf was hired to head the CrossFit nutrition certification program.

After bolting his breakfast, Brian returned home to prepare for the day's major task: recording a new webisode of the *UnScared Sports Show*. UnScared was the name of Brian's business, which functioned almost entirely within the CrossFit organization but was technically independent. The letters U-N-S-C-A-R-E-D were tattooed across Brian's fingers. His partner in the business was Doug Katona, who lived a few doors down from Brian and who arrived at Brian's house just after eight o'clock on this particular morning. Doug was forty-five years old but looked a full decade younger. A competitive cyclist, he trained with a mixture of bike rides and CrossFit workouts and, like Brian, he ate like a caveman.

The set of the *UnScared Sports Show* was an old couch in Brian's garage. Each new webisode was recorded by an unmanned camera and streamed live over the Internet before being archived on YouTube. In the middle of this day's thirty-minute program Isabella bum-rushed the couch and settled between Brian and Doug. They kept rolling. The topic of the day was nutrition. At one point Doug asked Brian to name the most common nutritional error he saw in athletes.

"People don't understand that once the volume and intensity of their training increase, they are not taking in enough fat," Brian said, accompanying his speech with a lot of hand gestures. "People do not understand how important that is. What we see when they start to take in more fat is that their nervous system starts to really buffer, they recover quicker, and the body becomes very fat-adaptive."

"What you want to do is train your body over time to access fat as a primary fuel source," Doug chimed in helpfully. He then turned back to his co-host. "So, what kind of fats are we talking about?"

Brian counted on his fingers. "Avocadoes," he began, "seeds, nuts (but not too many), anything with MCT's—medium-chain fats—especially coconut oil, olive oil, almond butter, and yes, even peanut butter, although I know a lot of the Paleo crowd is going to go fucking crazy on me for that."

Paleo purists do not eat peanuts because peanuts are technically legumes, not nuts, and while our Paleolithic ancestors ate nuts, supposedly they did not eat legumes. Brian Mackenzie was admittedly not a purist.

"Dude, if you can tolerate the peanuts, go for it," he told the camera. "If you can't, don't. Fuck it."

After the show, Brian cleared away some space in his garage and did his first workout of the day. The garage was not only his video set but also his gym. He did heavy sumo deadlifts for an hour with as much as 400 pounds while drawing motivation from an earsplitting soundtrack of Rage Against the Machine.

Dripping sweat, Brian made his way to the kitchen to prepare his second meal of the day, and the first of three smoothies. He blended coconut milk, a couple of huge handfuls of fresh spinach, three or four slices of raw bell pepper, a scoop of powdered greens, a few chunks of frozen banana, and a glob of peanut butter (fuck it) and drank the resulting viscous green concoction straight from the blender in huge gulps.

"Tastes like ass," he says.

Point of No Return

Paleo Diet creator Loren Cordain has no formal training as a paleobiologist or evolutionary biologist. A number of scientists with true expertise in these fields have stepped forward to discredit the core precepts of Cordain's diet. Perhaps the most celebrated Paleo Diet debunker is Christina Warinner, a biomolecular archeologist at the University of Zurich, who in the winter of 2013 delivered a TED talk called "Debunking the Paleo Diet." Warinner opened the talk with a clear declaration of her thesis, saying, "This version of the [Paleolithic] diet that is promoted in popular books, on TV, on self-help websites, and in the overwhelming majority of popular press has no basis in archeological reality." She then dismantled the theoretical foundation of the diet point by point.

In his book, Cordain advised people to get at least 50 percent of their daily calories from meat because our Paleolithic ancestors did the same. Warinner explained that this idea was based on flawed methods used to estimate meat intake from archeological evidence. The truth, she said, is that we don't really know how much meat the first humans and preceding hominids ate, but that it certainly varied greatly from place to place and was almost certainly very little in some places.

Cordain also warned people not to eat any grains or legumes because our Paleolithic ancestors did not. Warinner set him straight. "We have archeological evidence from at least 30,000 years ago—that's 20,000 years before the agricultural revolution—of stone tools that look like mortars and pestles that people used to grind up seeds and grain," she said, adding that new methods of extracting DNA from dental plaque (her own line of research) had recently revealed that both Neanderthals and Paleolithic peoples ate barley, beans, and tubers.

Four months after Warinner made these remarks, the *Proceedings of the National Academy of Sciences* published a set of four papers by researchers who had used these techniques to demonstrate that hominids living two and a half to three *million* years ago ate more grasses and grains than fruits and leaves.

Continuing to turn the screws, Warinner explained that nearly every food that our Paleolithic ancestors ate no longer exists today, and that virtually every food humans eat today is different from those eaten by our Paleolithic ancestors. "Let's take salads," she said. "That sounds like a really great Paleo Diet food. Except we've radically changed the ingredients to suit our needs. Wild lettuces contain a great deal of latex, which is indigestible and irritates our gastrointestinal system. It's bitter. The leaves are tough. We've domesticated them to be softer, to produce bigger leaves, to remove the latex and the bitterness, remove the spines that naturally grow on the leaves and stems of wild varieties, and make them tastier for us."

Paleolithic humans, it seems, *hated* their diet, and that's why they started a process of transforming it step by step into the modern diet.

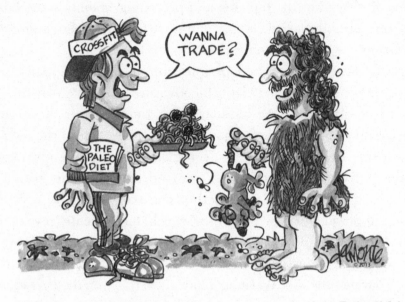

Actually, it would be more accurate to say that Paleolithic humans hated their *diets*—plural. For while Loren Cordain referred to an "original, universal diet" that all of our ancient ancestors shared, Warinner in her TED presentation said that in fact there were numerous Paleolithic human diets. She referred her audience's attention to a screen displaying an image of a model Paleo Diet breakfast taken from some Paleo website. "This looks like a delicious and nutritious breakfast," she said, "but it's not something a Paleolithic person would have had access to. First of all, the blueberries are from New England, the avocadoes are from Mexico, and the eggs are from China."

Beyond that, Warinner explained, the blueberries, avocadoes, and eggs that we enjoy today are quite unlike those eaten 20,000 years ago. Ancient avocadoes, for example, had only a couple of millimeters of edible fruit surrounding their pit.

The bottom line is that the Paleo Diet is not really what it claims to be. Nor does it do what it claims to do. Nutrition science has proven that saying "yes" to bacon and "no" to cheese, potatoes, and toast is not the most reliable way to attain maximum health.

Cordain claimed that a 50 percent meat diet was healthier than a diet with less meat. But a 2012 study by researchers at the Harvard School of Public Health found that the more red meat people ate, the sooner they died.

Paleo Diet proponents also claim that a diet lacking dairy is healthier than one that includes it. But in a 2010 review, Peter Elwood of Cardiff University in Wales reported that eating more dairy products was associated with a lower risk of heart disease, stroke, diabetes, and death by any cause.

Cordain and company argue as well that a diet excluding all grains is healthier than one that includes whole grains. But the massive National Institutes of Health–AARP Diet and Health Study, which tracked the disease and death rates of half a million men and women over nine years, found that those who ate the most whole grains were 22 percent less likely to die during the study period than were those who ate the least whole grains. The heaviest consumers of whole grains were also 29 percent less likely to develop heart disease.

Finally, Cordain has warned that eating legumes is certain to result in "serious [health] effects." But in a comprehensive review of past research on the role of legumes in cardiometabolic risk prevention, researchers at the University of Oran, Algeria reported that, in fact, legumes "provide health benefits, protecting against numerous diseases or disorders, such as coronary heart disease, diabetes, high blood pressure and inflammation."

The Paleo Diet cult's preferred way of dealing with such findings is to sweepingly dismiss them as tainted by food-industry influence. It is true that some nutrition research is biased by pecuniary pressures. But to paraphrase Abraham Lincoln, while you can corrupt some scientists some of the time, you cannot corrupt all of the scientists all of the time. I know a lot of nutrition scientists personally, and in my experience they take great pains to exclude bias from their work. If they don't always succeed, they at least try. The same cannot be said for the typical Paleo diet evangelist, who unashamedly expresses an urgent desire to preserve his belief in Paleo doctrine, a desire that is the very source of the defensive tactic of reflexively impugning the credibility of the scientists whose work discredits their treasured beliefs.

If Paleo Diet advocates are wrong about the dangers of not eating like a caveman, then they must also be wrong about the diet's founding premise, that the human body hasn't had enough time to adapt to post-Paleolithic additions to the diet. Again, science shows they are wrong indeed.

M. G. Thomas of University College London, for example, has shown that humans in northern Europe and in other areas where dairy farming was adopted in the early Neolithic period evolved to benefit from milk-drinking in a short period of time. The gene variant allowing a person to digest lactase (milk sugar) in adulthood went from being virtually nonexistent in northern Europeans 8,000 years ago, when dairy farming was introduced in the region, to being present in 80 percent of northern Europeans today.

The story with grains is similar. Anne Stone at Arizona State University has demonstrated that humans from populations with high-starch diets typically have more copies of a gene that regulates the production of amylase, an enzyme that aids starch digestion, than do individuals from populations with low-starch diets. So it appears that humans living in places where grain agriculture was adopted at the beginning of the Neolithic period evolved rather quickly to benefit from a grain-centered diet. This is hardly surprising, given the fact that our ancestors were eating a fair bit of wild grain more than two million years before.

The old concept of the genome as a fixed, deterministic "blueprint" for organisms, which Loren Cordain probably had in mind when he developed the Paleo Diet, has lately been replaced with a far more complex and dynamic model of genetics and evolution.

It is now understood that evolution—especially as it relates to dietary adaptation—is not always slow. Scientists have learned, for example, that organisms and species can evolve in response to environmental influences without *any* genetic changes through so-called epigenetic adjustments that turn existing genes "on" and "off."

The most conspicuous epigenetic adaptations are dietary. In a fascinating 1952 study, Bernard Squires reported finding that African Bushmen who had been on a high-starch European diet for three months produced four times as much salivary amylase as their tribesmen who remained on a traditional diet consisting almost entirely of meat. This finding suggests that late Paleolithic/ early Neolithic humans may have been able to adapt (epigenetically) to increased grain consumption quite easily, paving the way for subsequent genetic adaptations.

Wild Child

As a boy, Brian MacKenzie was a natural born hell-raiser. His parents did not know where the wild streak came from. Brian's father, Bruce, was a model of stability, a successful insurance broker who held the same job from the time Brian was born until the time he left the nest. His mother, Linell, stayed at home, keeping the house in order and her children fed (Brian had two younger siblings), spoiling everyone with affection. The family lived under the same roof in the pleasant Orange County City of Tustin throughout Brian's childhood.

As a toddler, Brian showed a strong disinclination to sit still. Classrooms were prisons to him. Always bent on the next adrenaline rush, Brian got into extreme sports—skateboarding, snowboarding, surfing—long before the X-Games brought them into the mainstream. He liked regular sports (soccer, water polo) too and excelled as a swimmer, specializing in the shortest, most balls-to-the-wall freestyle sprints. When he got a little older, Brian fell in with the punk crowd and started to do the things the punk crowd did. He drove like a maniac, got tattooed, and became known to the local constabulary. His mother worried, not without reason, that her firstborn would not live to see his eighteenth birthday, but Brian's interest in sports kept him from flying completely out of control.

Somehow Brian managed to graduate from high school. Not knowing what to do next, he drifted into taking classes at a local community college, where he also competed on the swim team, dragging himself out of bed for pre-dawn practices despite a flourishing late-night social life.

Around this time, Brian's dad got into powerlifting. Brian took a liking to it as well, and before long father and son were training together in the garage of the family home. Some of Brian's friends joined in, and Brian found himself serving as their de facto personal trainer, a role he enjoyed. Sniffing a potential calling, he dropped out of his first college, where he'd pursued general studies, and enrolled in another local two-year college where he was able to study exercise science. But although he liked the subject matter, a classroom was still a classroom and Brian struggled to stay motivated. So he quit—only to return for the next term, and then quit again, only to come back once more.

This recursive pattern continued for nine long years. There was even an abortive Navy stint somewhere in there. Brian was lost, searching, always moving—and going nowhere.

It was a spin class, of all things, that at last set Brian on the path he had been born to walk without ever knowing it. When the Spinning craze swept across America in the late 1990s, Brian got sucked in by the appeal of its hardcore intensity. He started going to classes in Newport Beach, where he and a like-minded spinner became friends. That new friend happened to be a triathlete, and he persuaded Brian to do an Ironman. Built to sprint twenty-five yards in a pool and to lift fantastic amounts of weight off the ground, Brian's body crumbled under the slow-drip punishment of heavy endurance training, but he liked it anyway. Swimming, cycling, and running for hours at a time was a different kind of challenge than whizzing down steep hills on a skateboard, yet it gave him a similar thrill—the thrill of spitting in the dragon's eye.

Brian soon moved up from triathlons to ultramarathons. The primal satisfaction he got from these all-day wilderness runs was even greater. But the training was even more destructive. Sixty to eighty miles a week of running left Brian's body feeling downright geriatric, and he kept getting injured.

Then he got an idea. Remembering how much better he had felt when he was hitting the weights hard, he went back to them, but modified his routine to support his running. He developed fast-paced, multimodal workouts that combined the durability-building benefit of Olympic-style weightlifting and the cardiovascular fitness boost of sprinting uphill. It worked. Brian discovered that his killer primal workouts delivered so much all-around fitness in so little time that he could drastically reduce his running volume without sacrificing performance. Fewer miles meant less wear and tear on his body, and fewer injuries. Brian's clients at Genetic Potential, a gym he'd opened, saw similar results.

In July 2007, a healthy Brian MacKenzie finished the Angels Crest 100-Mile Endurance Run. He did not win the race, but the thirty-three runners who finished ahead of him would have been shocked to learn how little running—and how many deadlifts—Brian had done to prepare for it.

It was a moment of epiphany. As he crossed the finish line, Brian already knew his next move. When he got home, he fired off a breathless email to Greg Glassman, founder of CrossFit. An eccentric former gymnast, Glassman had started CrossFit in 2000 to fill a void in the fitness landscape. CrossFit workouts are unbridled multidisciplinary suffer-fests similar to those that Brian had come up with independently. A typical workout is "Cindy" (every CrossFit workout has a name), which requires the participant to complete as many rounds of five pull-ups, ten push-ups, and fifteen body weight squats as possible in twenty minutes. CrossFit workouts like Cindy have been known to cause rhabdomyolosis, a potentially life-threatening condition where the liver is flooded with toxins released from damaged muscles. Brian had tried CrossFit and, of course, he loved it.

By 2007 CrossFit was a juggernaut, and Brian saw an opportunity. In his message to Glassman (whom CrossFitters refer to exclusively as "Coach," one of several cultish behaviors of the tribe), Brian explained what his new, CrossFit-inspired method of training had done for him and for the endurance athletes he trained. He invited Glassman to entertain a vision of CrossFit infiltrating the gigantic and ever-growing endurance market. Five hours later Brian received a reply.

"You've piqued my interest."

Brian was given a tryout. Glassman tasked him to create a one-off clinic that would present his methods to interested Cross-Fitters. If Glassman approved of the material, Brian would be set loose to do as many more clinics as there was demand for. Brian nailed the audition and with Coach's coveted blessing, CrossFit Endurance was born. The franchise now produces more than 100 clinics a year and continues to grow. Brian no longer leads most of the clinics himself but has hired ten staff coaches who oversee an even larger number of assistant coaches who manage a still greater number of interns. Revenues for the operation are estimated to exceed two million dollars annually.

When CrossFit Endurance was just getting off the ground, Brian attended a talk by CrossFit's in-house Paleo diet guru, Robb Wolf. He was impressed. The man knew his material. Everything Wolf said made perfect sense. Words and phrases like "lectins" and "protease inhibitors" rolled off his tongue with the greatest of ease. Wolf explained that lectins were "dangerous" proteins in grains which the protease inhibitors also present in grains shepherded "intact" through the intestinal walls and deep into the body, where they caused "serious problems."

Wolf's book, *The Paleo Solution*, went into greater detail and supplemented the nitty-gritty biology with a goodly amount of testimonial—and salesmanship. In a hair-raising first chapter, Wolf described how a tragically misguided youthful foray into vegetarianism had nearly killed him, resulting in high blood pressure, high triglycerides, high cholesterol, colitis, nearly constant pain throughout his body, insomnia, debilitating depression, and extreme weight loss.

"I literally wanted to die, but I was too chicken to do the deed," he wrote.

Then, just in the nick of time, Wolf discovered the Paleo Diet. His first Paleo meal was a rack of ribs and a salad. It cured him instantly. *Instantly.*

"This book could save your life," Wolf told his readers.

Like Robb Wolf, Brian Mackenzie had been raised on a typical American diet of breakfast cereal, sandwiches, and pasta. His favorite food was pizza, which he ate at least once a week. Upon discovering the Paleo Diet, Brian got rid of all that "crap" and started eating the way he does today. Unlike Wolf, however, Brian was not cured instantly. For the first three or four weeks he was miserable. Paleo people call this malaise the "ketogenic flu"—a grab bag of symptoms including headaches, moodiness, and lethargy that attend a sudden and drastic reduction in carbohydrate consumption. Having weaned himself off booze years earlier, Brian deemed the ketogenic flu no worse than "the horrors," and the eventual rewards were even greater.

When he came out the other side, Brian discovered that his immune system was impenetrable—he never got sick anymore. Even better, his training became supercharged. He began to recover from hard workouts as though he were eighteen years old again. Meanwhile, he dropped body fat like ballast from a hot-air balloon. On top of all that, his energy and mental focus no longer dipped at mid-afternoon.

These results may not be typical. A 2013 study reported that after ten weeks on the indiscriminately meat-centered Paleo program, forty-three healthy adults showed significantly increased levels of LDL ("bad") cholesterol. Athletes who go Paleo often complain that their training is sabotaged by the diet's parsimonious supply of carbohydrates. But Brian MacKenzie felt nothing less than reborn on the Paleo path.

"It's the best thing that's ever happened to me," he told me.

Birds of a Feather

Within a month of being uploaded to YouTube, Christina Warinner's "Debunking the Paleo Diet" presentation had attracted more than two thousand viewer comments. Most of them were angry retorts posted by followers of the Paleo Diet.

"This is just pure vegan propaganda horse shit," wrote Ryan Lewis.

Others addressed Warinner directly. "I fail to see the debunking," wrote Matthew Powell, "and you didn't really have a solid grasp of paleo/primal ideology. Let us also not neglect the large amount of assumption and speculation in the field of archeology."

Mike Parker was one of many commenters who echoed Mr. Powell's idea that, despite its title, the speech was fundamentally supportive of Paleo doctrine. "Her whole talk is basically just a nice elaboration and clarification of paleo diets, not a debunking of their main ideas," he wrote.

John Martin was more blunt, writing, "Her presentation contradicts the title of her talk. What bullshit!"

Richard Lawson drew attention to a particular perceived contradiction. "She stated that our bodies are not designed to eat meat," Lawson complained, "but later stated that our paleo ancestors did eat meat. What?"

Others invoked the much abused straw-man defense. "She defines 'paleo' to mean something ridiculous and then proceeds to pick it apart," wrote Jason Brown. "It's a straw man argument."

There is a desperateness to these defenses which seems to suggest that Warinner's critics did not simply believe but *wanted* to believe the Paleo Diet was the One True Way to eat for maximum health. Indeed, given the scientific refutation of the diet's premise and benefit claims, *only* someone who wanted to believe in them could. Who would want to hold these beliefs and why? We get a clue from a review of the first names of the angry critics quoted above: Ryan, Matthew, Mike, Jason, Richard, John.

That's right: all men.

Although hard data on the makeup of the Paleo Diet cult are scant, it appears to be a decidedly male phenomenon. Christina Warinner made reference to this imbalance in her presentation.

"The diet does seem primarily targeted at men," she said. "If you look at advertisements and descriptions you see virile caveman-like images, slogans like 'Live primal!', and lots of red meat."

You don't have to have a PhD in anthropology to know that the caveman ethos appeals to masculine identity. The stereotype of the spear-wielding primeval antelope-slayer is generally more attractive to men than it is to women. The Paleo Diet is hardly unique in having a gender imbalance among its members. Nearly 60 percent of vegetarians, for example, are women. Many vegetarians believe that *their* diet is the One True Way. Mainstream nutrition science doesn't support this notion either. Like Paleo dieters, hardcore vegetarians *want* to believe that their way is the One True Way. Something about not eating animals appeals to a disposition—perhaps one of compassion—that is more common in women than in men.

Gender is not the only factor that informs people's attractions to particular diet cults. Politics is another. Politically liberal women *and* men are 40 percent more likely to be vegetarian than are moderates and conservatives.

Believing in a diet (or anything else) because one wants to believe in it does not automatically make one an idiot. Many of the angry critics who commented on the video of Christina Warinner's presentation were smart enough to admit that it just isn't possible to eat today as our ancestors ate twenty thousand years ago. Yet they still insisted on defending what they called the "essence" of the diet.

"She really hasn't debunked anything at all," wrote Rob Nash. "The essence of the Paleo Diet is to eat a wide variety of seasonal foods in their whole form. The Paleo Diet today is an adaptation based on what is available today."

This defense is no less desperate than the others. For if Loren Cordain had wanted to do nothing more than advocate eating "a wide variety of seasonal foods in their whole form," presumably he would have done that. But he didn't. He advocated eating *just like a primordial hunter-gatherer.* And he was smart to do so, in a sense. If Cordain had merely advocated eating a wide variety of seasonal foods in their whole form, his book would have flopped. Not sexy enough. It was the idea of eating just like a primordial hunter-gatherer that got millions of folks like Rob Nash excited.

The caveman fantasy is appealing not only to masculine self-image but also to certain masculine cultures. As I mentioned earlier, the Paleo Diet is especially popular among some types of athletes, who perhaps identify with the physicality of the caveman stereotype. The more "primal" the sport, the more Paleo dieters you'll find in it. The macho gestalt of the bodybuilding culture and the outdoorsy ethos of the ultrarunning tribe, for example, are better aligned with the Paleo fantasy than are the urban vibe of basketball and the hoity-toity culture of golf. But no athletic community has embraced the Paleo Diet more enthusiastically than the cult of CrossFit.

The convergence of CrossFit and the Paleo Diet was inevitable. A similar spirit animates both cults. There's a raw quality to each that confers the same sense of superiority upon those who embrace it: the kind that says, "I reject this artificial modern life!" If you're attracted to the Paleo Diet, you're bound to have a weakness for CrossFit, and vice versa. In his book, Robb Wolf even argued that CrossFit workouts somehow mimic the fight-or-flight lifestyle of our Paleolithic ancestors and thus fit our genes in much the same way the Paleo Diet does.

Mainstream science once again begs to differ. Outside of Loren Cordain himself, exercise physiologists do not believe that CrossFit is intrinsically more effective or natural than other forms of exercise. There's no evidence that a person who works hard at Zumba or triathlon can't get just as fit as the most hardcore CrossFitter.

It is neither a shared basis in truth nor superior effectiveness that links CrossFit and the Paleo Diet. The men and women (but mostly men) who get into both of these practices are not smarter than other people. They're just more susceptible to that back-to-the-jungle gestalt—suckers for the romantic vision of chasing wild boars with slingshots, which is all the more romantic when one entertains it while eating a Waldorf salad (an actual recipe in *The Paleo Diet*) at a chic bistro on the strip. CrossFitters who embrace the Paleo Diet and Paleo eaters who get into CrossFit like to believe that *reason* led them to where they have arrived. But in fact the pipeline between these two cults has nothing to do with truth and everything to do with personal disposition, culture, and community.

A Man in His Element

After a lunch of vegetable salad, beef tri-tip, and steamed broccoli at another favorite local restaurant, Brian MacKenzie settled down in front of his computer back home to write some workouts for a few of the seven or eight clients he trained remotely. While Brian's coaching services were much in demand, he didn't have time to train more than a handful of clients properly and he hardly needed the money he turned away.

At two o'clock Brian called his girlfriend and unofficial client, Erin Carfaro, a gold medalist in rowing at the Beijing Olympics who was currently competing in Germany with her teammates before heading to London for the 2012 Summer Games (where she would win a second gold medal). During the chat, Erin confessed to having eaten some sort of German noodles at a team meal. Brian gently chastised her for the lapse.

After hanging up, Brian changed clothes for his second workout of the day: a CrossFit workout called Helen. He turned up the volume on some Tool and made his way to the back patio, where he completed three rounds of the following as quickly as possible: 400 meters on a rowing machine, ten kettlebell swings with a fifty-four-pound weight, and twelve pull-ups. Early in the workout, a blister burst on his right hand. He kept going. Blood flowed and the open wound became increasingly painful. By the time he got to the last set of pull-ups, he could barely hold on to the bar. He kept going. When he stopped the clock (at eight minutes exactly, one of his better times for the session) his palm was a gory mess.

Brian rounded out his day's nutrition with another smoothie and, a couple of hours later, dinner: a one-pound hamburger topped with bacon sitting on a spinach salad with steamed broccoli, sliced bell peppers, and carrots. His evening was spent packing. In the morning he would fly to Columbus, Ohio, where a couple of his clients would compete in a CrossFit Games regional championship. On the heels of this excursion there would be trips to Germany, the East Coast, the San Francisco Bay Area, Los Angeles (for the 2012 CrossFit Games), and finally London, for the Olympics.

Fifteen years earlier, before he had found his true calling, Brian could not have imagined he would end up where he was on this flawless spring day. He had recently appeared on the cover of *Competitor* magazine. In Ohio tomorrow he would be mobbed for autographs and photos. He was dating a world-class athlete. He had his own book coming out. He was a regular dinner companion of Greg Glassman, Coach, the founder of CrossFit. He wouldn't trade his life for anyone's.

The Myth of Rational Choice

Followers of all healthy-diet cults like to believe that their particular choice of diet was made rationally. As they see it, they just looked at the facts and saw what everyone ought to see: that the Paleo Diet (or vegetarianism, or gluten-free eating, or whatever) was undeniably superior to other diets. But these folks are fooling themselves. People don't choose diets: diets choose people. Dig into the personality and life history of any diet-cult member and you will find at least one obvious emotional or social basis for the match. Whether it's gender or parentage or politics or geography or some other factor, there's always some identity-based source of *willingness* to believe what a particular diet cult would have one believe. This isn't just my observation; a number of recent studies have demonstrated that people reflexively alter their dietary beliefs and practices—sometimes from one moment to the next—to conform to those of peer groups.

Often it's as simple as who your friends are. Perhaps you are bitten by the CrossFit bug, and before you know it you're making CrossFit friends, going where other CrossFitters go, dressing like them, talking like them, reading what they read, listening to the music they like, and, of course, eating like them.

5

The Suck-It-Up Diet

There are some people who would never move to a city with harsh winters. The perfect job might await them in Buffalo or Minneapolis, but the inescapable fact of January would render the opportunity a nonstarter. There are others who couldn't be persuaded to relocate to a city known for its sweltering summers. No conceivable pay increase could entice such a person to trade Portland or Flagstaff for Houston or Phoenix. Still others draw the line at places they consider too dull, or too dangerous, too backward, or too godless.

And then there's Brandy Alles, who vows she would never move to an area that lacked a Weight Watchers center. So far she's been as good as her word. When she was twenty-eight years old, Brandy, then residing in her native Atlanta, was offered an attractive job as a marketing coordinator in Charlotte, North Carolina. She searched online and discovered that Charlotte was home to a few Weight Watchers centers. She accepted the offer.

Brandy rented an apartment close to one center and attended her first meeting there before she had even taken up full-time residence in her new home. Brandy hated to go more than a couple of weeks without a meeting. Weight Watchers was a lifeline for her.

"I will probably be on Weight Watchers for the rest of my life," she told me matter-of-factly.

Most people who become severely overweight are reared by parents with weight problems of their own, but Brandy Alles is an exception. Her father owned a chain of health clubs in the Atlanta area. Her mother too had a passion for fitness and healthy living. Brandy and her siblings were served vegetables with each nightly home-cooked meal and there was always an abundance of fresh fruit in the house. Brandy did not inherit her parents' love of physical activity, however. She quit school sports (until then her only source of exercise) after middle school. Worse, she developed a sweet tooth and a slow metabolism that were somehow lacking in the rest of the family. By the time Brandy got her driver's license, she was already full-figured.

In college, Brandy's figure got even fuller. She gained more than fifty pounds at Brigham Young University, thanks to a diet of cafeteria meals supplemented with snacks from vending machines. A tendency toward emotional eating didn't help matters. Brandy tried her best to live in denial of her steadily increasing weight by avoiding mirrors and scales. But deep inside she was not fooling herself. In fact, she was freaking out. Every once in a while, her panic broke to the surface in the form of a headlong plunge into some weight-loss diet. She tried all of them: Atkins, South Beach, Jenny Craig, NutriSystem, Sugar Busters, a couple of juice cleanses, Slimfast, and even the Kellogg's breakfast cereal diet. Each time she lost a few pounds but then grew frustrated with onerous restrictions, relentless hunger, and unmet expectations and quit the diet after several weeks, ultimately gaining back all the weight she had lost plus a little extra.

In the fall of 2009, Brandy went in for her annual physical. Her physician took Brandy through the usual routine of stethoscope and blood-pressure cuff and tongue depressor. But when all that was done, the doctor suddenly departed from the familiar script.

"We need to have a serious discussion," she said.

Brandy swallowed hard. She knew what was coming. Brandy was informed that she weighed 241 pounds. Her body mass index classified her as borderline obese. Her blood pressure and her "bad" and total cholesterol numbers were high and had risen sharply since her last physical. If she didn't change course soon, the doctor said, Brandy would have to start taking medications to stave off her inevitable first stroke or heart attack. She was twenty-six.

Upon returning home, Brandy told her roommate, Ashley, what had happened. Ashley had recently lost thirty pounds for her wedding on Weight Watchers. She had never pushed Weight Watchers on Brandy, but it now seemed almost wrong not to extend an invitation.

"Come to a meeting," Ashley said. "Just one. You don't have to sign up. I won't pressure you. You can decide for yourself."

Brandy had previously lacked any interest in joining Weight Watchers, despite her friend's success. It seemed too great a commitment—or perhaps too public a forum for failure. But her recent scare had knocked down that barrier. She felt she had nothing to lose. Brandy accompanied Ashley to a meeting, where she was struck by the supportiveness of the environment. It was like a sisterhood. She signed up.

Strength in Numbers

Weight Watchers was founded in 1963 by a Brooklyn homemaker named Jean Nidetch. At that time America's obesity crisis was just beginning, and Nidetch was an early victim of "too much meat and too little exercise," as she put it. She tried various fad diets without success before losing twenty pounds at a diet clinic. But keeping the weight off was a struggle. Nidetch had a hunch that a little social support would make a big difference, so she formed a support group with friends who were also trying to lose weight. They met once a week. That sisterhood became Weight Watchers, which is now the world's leading provider of weight-loss services.

The Weight Watchers program is based on what the organization calls the four scientifically proven pillars of weight loss: healthy eating, exercise, behavior modification, and social support. The support piece is the one that Weight Watchers hangs its hat on, but since 1997 the organization has perhaps been best known for its points system. Now branded the PointsPlus program, this system assigns a point value to every kind of food under the sun and allots to each dieter an individual daily points quota to ensure she does not overeat. There are no forbidden foods, but high-calorie foods carry a lot of points, so dieters cannot eat much of them without exceeding their daily quota.

Weight Watchers is more than a successful company with a loyal customer base: it is a full-fledged subculture. Longtime Weight Watchers members develop a strong devotion to the organization that is often expressed as a fierce defensiveness. Peer pressure is the fuel that now powers the Weight Watchers social dynamic. Happy members routinely exploit social bonds to discourage struggling members from quitting. The public weigh-ins at meetings bear some resemblance to the shaming rituals of bona fide cults. Many members exhibit a sort of fetishistic attachment to the points system. A *New York Times* article once described this system as having a "cult-like following."

A few former members have come right out and labeled Weight Watchers a cult. These accusations may say more about the accusers than the accused. While Weight Watchers certainly qualifies as a diet cult, it is not a cult in the dictionary sense any more than the Rotary Club is. The features that give the Weight Watchers community a vaguely cult-like character have not harmed anyone and they are the very things that make it effective for people like Brandy Alles.

A handful of studies have found that the Weight Watchers program compares favorably to other weight-loss methods. A British study pitted Weight Watchers against a clinical weight-loss program administered by the national health-care system. Over the course of one year, overweight individuals assigned to Weight Watchers lost more than twice as much weight as those who dieted under a doctor's care.

But to conclude from these findings that Weight Watchers is a more effective way to lose weight than following a doctor's advice would be akin to saying that buying two Powerball tickets is a more effective way to win the lottery than buying one ticket. Most people don't win the lottery regardless of how many tickets they buy. Likewise, people who join Weight Watchers are as likely to fail to achieve *permanent* weight loss as are people who try by other means.

In 2008 scientists at Drexel University studied long-term weight-loss maintenance in a large population of Weight Watchers "lifetime members." All of the more than 900 individuals (the vast majority of them women) included in the study had succeeded in meeting their original weight-loss goal through the Weight Watchers program. They were the cream of the crop—the program's most successful clients. The Drexel researchers tracked the weight of these individuals for five years after they had attained their goal. At the end of this period only 16 percent of them remained at their goal weight, and only half had maintained even 5 percent of their original weight loss.

Brandy Alles lost a surprising seven pounds in her first week on Weight Watchers. But what really bowled her over was how easy it was. She felt no hunger or cravings. Something was different this time. Somehow Brandy *knew* she would succeed. On all of her past diets, she only now realized, she had known deep inside that she would fail. The camaraderie of the meetings was the main thing she liked about Weight Watchers, but the program's bullshit-free approach to diet also appealed to her. The plan had no real shtick. It was simple, straightforward, and commonsensical. It suddenly occurred to Brandy that, despite having been raised by a couple of health nuts and having read innumerable diet books, she had never acquired a *common sense* for healthy eating until she found Weight Watchers.

Before Weight Watchers, Brandy ate a majority of her meals at fast-food restaurants—Arby's and Taco Bell being her favorites. She indulged her sweet tooth without restraint, gobbling ice cream, chocolate, and pastries whenever the desire struck. On Weight Watchers, Brandy restricted her restaurant habit to one or two meals a week. She ate fat-free yogurt or low-sugar oatmeal for breakfast, low-fat sandwiches and Lean Cuisine entrees for lunch, fruit and nuts for snacks, and lean meats and fish with heaping piles of veggies for dinner. The foods changed a bit from day to day, but one thing stayed the same: Brandy never exceeded her points limit.

After that magical first week, Brandy continued to lose weight rapidly for several months. Eventually, though, her progress slowed. When that happened she took the advice of her Weight Watchers meeting leader and added exercise to her regimen, and the pounds started flying off again. She began with walking, advanced to jogging, and then ventured into Bikram yoga, workout videos, kickboxing, you name it.

Two years into her Weight Watchers journey, Brandy leveled off at 141 pounds. She had lost exactly 100 pounds. At her next physical exam Brandy's doctor did not recognize her—not in the sense of, "Wow, you look different," but in the sense that she believed Brandy was a stranger she had never before set eyes on.

That felt good, but it was another incident that really knocked Brandy upside the head with a full sense of her achievement. She was shopping at Home Depot with Ashley, the roommate who had introduced her to Weight Watchers. They were passing through the lawn and garden section when they came upon a stack of fifty-pound bags of rocks.

"Look at that," Ashley said, pointing at the rocks. "You used to have two of those bags strapped to your body! I'll bet you can't even pick one of them up."

Brandy could not resist the challenge. She squatted down and hoisted a bag—it wasn't easy, but she managed to get herself fully upright with the rocks clutched to her chest. She then set down the rocks and tried scooping two bags into her arms, but they might as well have been cemented to the floor. It was almost impossible to believe that she had carried a living equivalent of that immovable mass on her body every day for years. Equally unfathomable was the damage it must have been doing to her. *Never again*, Brandy swore to herself. *Never again.*

Follow the Losers

People like Brandy Alles are rare. You're almost as likely to meet someone who has been struck by lightning twice as you are to encounter a person who has lost more than 40 percent of her peak body weight and kept it all off longer than a year. Such people not only deserve to be congratulated, but they are also a potentially valuable resource for the millions of other men and women who dream of accomplishing a similar transformation. In a world where almost nothing that is done with the intent of permanent weight loss works, folks like Brandy are living examples of what does.

Yet until fairly recently, obesity researchers showed little interest in mining this resource. It did not cross their minds that they might learn something from everyday folks who had already solved for themselves what the scientists sought to solve for everyone with fancy theories deduced from biological evidence.

Most studies in the field of obesity research are *interventional* in nature. An interventional study is one in which a researcher comes up with a theoretically plausible method of weight loss and then tries it out on a group of volunteers and compares the results against the (non-)results of untreated control subjects. The opposite of this approach is the *observational* study, where a researcher with a little humility gathers together a bunch of people like Brandy Alles and asks, "So, how did you do it?"

Interventional studies have their place in obesity research, but they don't necessarily bear much relevance to the real world. If a scientist decides that eating less fat is the secret to permanent weight loss and he puts volunteers on a low-fat diet and the average subject loses a few pounds, whereas volunteers who continue to eat as they've been eating lose no weight—well, that's great, but we're still a long way from knowing whether this finding can make a real difference outside the ivory tower. And time has taught us that such findings make no difference. Over the past several decades, scientists have identified dozens of dietary manipulations that yield statistically significant amounts of short-term weight loss in clinical environments, and meanwhile the general population has become fatter and fatter.

It wasn't until 1994 that a pair of scientists with a bit of humility hit upon the idea that the true secret to permanent weight loss might actually be whatever it was that the few achievers of significant long-term weight loss were doing. Rena Wing, a behavioral psychologist at Brown University, and James Hill, a pediatrician at the University of Colorado, recognized that most dieters who lost weight, including most people who lost weight as subjects in clinical studies, eventually regained it. Wing and Hill wanted to find out how those rare achievers of lasting weight loss defied the odds. They founded the National Weight Control Registry and invited anyone who had lost at least thirty pounds and kept the weight off at least one year to join. Thousands did. Wing and Hill and their colleagues gathered tons of data from these "successful losers" and sifted it for common patterns.

As you might expect, the collaborators were most interested in learning what these people ate. They assumed, as we all do, that the secret to permanent weight loss was a certain way of eating. Wing and Hill expected to find that the majority of successful losers shared some type of common diet. Perhaps it was the low-fat thing that worked for them. Or maybe meat avoidance was the trick. Or possibly sugar restriction. Whatever the secret turned out to be, Wing and Hill could then turn around and promote it to others as truly the most effective diet for weight loss.

Nine years after the National Weight Control Registry was created, James Hill summarized what he and Rena Wing had learned about the diets of successful losers at a public symposium hosted by Kaiser Permanente.

"We could not find factors common to the diets used by registry participants for weight loss," Hill said.

That's right: there was no pattern. No key. No secret. While all of the NWCR members owed their weight loss to dietary changes of some kind, these changes lacked any consistency. They were all over the map. Some people found success through commercial weight-loss programs like Weight Watchers. Others did it completely on their own. Some used low-fat, high-carb diets. Others used high-fat, low-cab diets. Some lost weight through liquid diets and weight-loss supplements. Others got slimmer by eliminating supplements and other "fake foods" from their diet. Having expected to unearth the single most effective diet for weight loss in the real world, Wing and Hill were instead stunned to discover that there was no such diet.

This does not mean that what a person eats is completely irrelevant to weight loss. There are some important differences between the diets of successful losers and the diet of the average American. For example, successful losers eat more vegetables and fewer sweets. But within the population of successful losers, there is just as much individual diversity in eating patterns as there is outside of it. There is no general formula that we can point to and urge everyone to imitate. As helpful as it might be to say, "If you want to lose weight, you *must* eat this and not that," we cannot do so in good faith. The registry members have taught us that there are more ways to lose weight than there are ways to win a chess game.

Meanwhile, the world marches on as though eating a certain way (but which way?) really were the secret to permanent weight loss. Bariatric scientists continue to search for the weight-loss diet that ends obesity once and for all. Nutrition gurus continue to promote branded weight-loss diets as superior to all others. Overweight men and women continue to hope they are able to identify the One True Way to lose weight among the many options. But they're all barking up the wrong tree, because the particular diet that helps one person achieve permanent weight loss is likely to prove unsustainable for another person.

Was the National Weight Control Registry then a complete waste of time? No. To say that no specific diet is the true secret to permanent weight loss is not to say that there is no secret. In fact, there is a secret—it just has nothing to do with what a person eats. The true secret to weight loss is revealed through a few key behaviors that are shared by nearly all of the men and women who achieve major permanent weight loss. Rena Wing and James Hill may have come up empty-handed in their search for a diet common to NWCR members, but they did manage to identify three specific things that successful losers do—and most dieters don't—that serve as clues to what it *really* takes to lose weight permanently.

One of them is self-weighing. The bathroom scale has long been an object of controversy in the dieting community. One camp has discouraged frequent weigh-ins on the grounds that they foster an unhealthy obsession with fast results. Others, including Weight Watchers, have taken the commonsense position that if your goal is to lose weight, you ought to weigh yourself. The study of successful losers has shown that the Weight Watchers camp has it right. In 2007, Wing and Hill tracked self-weighing habits and actual changes in weight among 3,000 registry members. On average, the subjects whose frequency of self-weighing decreased during that year regained almost four times more weight than did those whose frequency of self-weighing increased.

Wing and Hill concluded that consistent self-weighing "may help individuals maintain their successful weight loss by allowing them to catch weight gains before they escalate and make behavior changes to prevent additional weight gain."

A second behavior that is common among successful losers and seems to be linked to their success is eating monotonously. Although individual registry members eat very differently from one another, they share a pattern of eating a smaller variety of foods than the typical fat person does. Nutrition scientists use a standard tool called the Health Habits and History Questionnaire to assess the variety in a person's diet. There are seven categories of foods in the tool, ranging from fruit to fats, oils, and sweets. You might expect that successful losers would eat a greater-than-average variety of foods in "good" categories such as fruits and less variety in "bad" categories such as fats, oils, and sweets. But in a 2005 study, Wing and Hill discovered that NWCR members consumed less variety in *all seven food categories* than did members of a control group.

The scientists speculated that eating the same foods and meals over and over helped dieters keep their calorie intake within acceptable limits. When you think about it, this idea makes sense. Any time your diet strays into less familiar territory, the results are less predictable than they are when you stick with what is already proven to work for you.

In addition to eating a smaller variety of all categories of foods from day to day, successful losers vary their eating habits less from weekdays to weekends and between the holiday season and the rest of the year. This might not sound like a huge deal, but research has shown that nearly all weight gain occurs on weekends and during the holiday season. The average American gains approximately one pound between Thanksgiving and New Year's Day and never loses it. This accounts for the bulk of the long-term weight gain that the average American experiences during the first twenty-five years of adulthood.

The remainder is accounted for by changes in the way people eat between Friday night and Sunday afternoon. Most people maintain a steady weight during the week but gain weight on weekends. The problem is not that they eat more of the same foods on their days of rest. Rather, they indulge in foods and drinks that they do not consume during the week: buttered popcorn at the movie theater, a couple of drinks with a heavy restaurant dinner, pancakes for breakfast on a leisurely Sunday morning. In contrast, successful losers don't slack off their dietary rules—whatever they may be—on weekends. They eat the same limited variety of foods on Saturday as they do on Wednesday.

A third behavioral habit of successful losers that points toward the true secret to permanent weight loss is exercise. Ninety percent of NWCR members used a combination of dietary changes and exercise to achieve their initial weight loss. We're not talking about a small amount of exercise, either. Wing and Hill monitored a sample of members and found that on average they burned 2,621 calories per week through structured physical activity. That's enough activity to burn off almost forty pounds in one year.

While the lion's share of NWCR members' initial weight loss is credited to diet, exercise does more than diet to prevent the reversal of those losses. In fact, physical activity is the single strongest predictor of weight regain in persons who have lost more than thirty pounds. Those who exercise a lot make up the small minority that stays skinny. Those who stop exercising altogether almost invariably gain back every ounce.

At first blush, the three key behaviors of successful losers—frequent self-weighing, dietary consistency, and lots of exercise—may appear unconnected. On closer inspection, though, the behaviors reveal themselves as indicators of a high level of *motivation* to lose weight. Daily self-weighing may be a bit obsessive, but who's more likely to succeed in losing weight: one who is obsessed with losing weight, or one who is not? Eating the same foods seven days a week, twelve months a year takes discipline—the sort of discipline you might expect from someone who is utterly determined not to fail. Most dieters exercise little, if they exercise at all. People who are *serious* about losing weight, like Brandy Alles (on her umpteenth try), do.

If the National Weight Control Registry has taught us anything, it has taught us that a person who is sufficiently motivated to lose weight is bound to succeed regardless of which diet she chooses to follow. By the same token, a person who is less than fully determined to lose weight is all but doomed to fail regardless of which diet he selects. There is no weight-loss system that teaches dieters to weigh themselves every day, eat the same meals every day, do tons of exercise, and choose their own set of diet changes. Successful losers develop these habits on their own because they would sooner perish than fail. Sure, the habits are helpful, but it's the motivation behind them that matters. The cliché is true: where there's a will, there's a way.

Most people assume that successful weight loss is not about the will but the way. They believe that dropping pounds depends on acquiring knowledge of the "correct" way to lose weight. Not so. The average third-grader possesses all the information that is required to lose weight. Nothing could be simpler.

Some years ago Richard Muller, a physics professor at UC Berkeley, decided that he needed to lose weight. He approached the problem like a physicist—that is, mathematically. Muller calculated that he ate 650 calories in his standard lunch. He then stopped eating it. He lost thirty pounds in two months.

It does not take a great deal of knowledge to figure out that eliminating a meal from one's day will yield weight loss. But it takes a high level of motivation to follow through on the idea. This is true of any path by which one might choose to pursue weight loss. Most paths are simple in principle and hard in practice. Few dieters fail for lack of knowledge. They fail because knowing does not guarantee doing.

Motivation is different than willpower. Think of willpower as a component of your brain's hardware—fixed and unchanging. Motivation is more like a piece of software or content that your brain uses but is not part of the brain. Motivators serve to activate willpower. Without motivation, having a lot of willpower is useless because there's no way to activate it. But motivation is equally useless without willpower, because in that case there's nothing to access. Since willpower is relatively fixed, if a person lacks the willpower to suck it up and do what it takes to lose weight, she's screwed. But if it's only motivation that a person lacks, there's hope. It is always possible to plug a better and stronger new motivator into the brain. Happily, the evidence suggests that most people have all the willpower they need to lose weight and that what separates the successful losers from the failures is motivation.

Both willpower and motivation are seated in the brain. Brain-imaging studies confirm that there is something fundamentally different going on between the ears of successful dieters. Rena Wing and James Hill have been involved in a couple of studies where people who were currently overweight, people who had never been overweight, and people who had lost weight were exposed to food temptations while having their brains scanned.

The resulting images revealed that successful losers experienced just as much food temptation as overweight persons (and more temptation than people who had never been overweight), but they also exhibited greater activity in the frontal lobes, the brain regions responsible for impulse inhibition.

While intriguing, these glances inside the skulls of successful losers do not tell us whether innate willpower or acquired motivation is responsible for long-term weight-loss maintenance. Either willpower or motivation could account for the higher level of activity in impulse-inhibition areas of the brain. To answer the question definitively, we must look at other evidence.

The scientific word for willpower is *self-control*. Psychologists have created standardized questionnaires that they use to measure individual self-control. The accuracy of these scales has been validated through tests, including a famous one where subjects were left alone in a room with food temptations under orders not to touch them. Longitudinal studies have revealed that children with strong self-control get better grades and become adults who are more likely to hold high-paying jobs, avoid hospitals, stay married, and raise children in a two-parent home, and are less likely to go to jail and—yes—become overweight. So it's pretty darn important.

But there's one thing that people with strong self-control (or willpower) do no better than people with weak self-control: diet. While men and women with a lot of innate willpower are less likely to become overweight in the first place, studies have shown that people with strong self-control who do become overweight are only a teensy bit more successful in their dieting efforts than are people with weaker self-control. This finding tells us that successful weight loss probably has more to do with present motivation than with underlying willpower.

Further evidence comes from another common characteristic of successful losers. Ninety percent of National Weight Control

Registry members report having failed in at least one attempt to lose weight before ultimately succeeding. A majority failed more than once. Brandy Alles, who abandoned at least a dozen diets before succeeding with Weight Watchers, is typical in this regard. Naturally, if lack of innate willpower were the reason people like Brandy failed with diets, then they could never succeed. The fact that today's successful losers are yesterday's failed dieters is very strong evidence that motivation—not will-power—is the key.

Motivation has been studied explicitly within the National Weight Control Registry. Eighty-two percent of NWCR members say that they were more committed to making behavioral changes in their final, successful attempt to lose weight than they had been in previous attempts. An equal percentage say they exercised more and 63 percent used a "stricter" dietary approach than in past efforts. They didn't necessarily try anything different. They just tried harder.

Eighty-three percent of NWCR members are able to identify a specific trigger for their breakthrough weight-loss attempt. All of these triggers are motivational in nature. The most common ones are experiencing an adverse medical event (23 percent), reaching an all-time high in weight (21.3 percent), and seeing oneself in a photograph or mirror and being horrified (12.7 percent). Interest-ingly, the medical trigger predicts the greatest success. Those who are motivated to lose weight by a surprise diagnosis or a sudden health setback lose 12.5 percent more weight and gain back 33 percent less over the next two years.

Here again, Brandy's story is typical. Her frightening doc-tor's appointment made her feel differently about losing weight than she ever had before. Fearing for her life, she started Weight Watchers with a resolve that had been missing in her past attempts to lose weight. Brandy herself gives most of the credit to Weight Watchers, but as we've seen, the vast majority of people who try

Weight Watchers do not get the results she did, while others are just as likely to succeed on different diets.

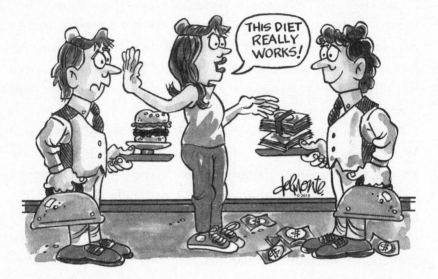

The trouble with motivation is that it's difficult to control and exploit. A nationwide program that trained physicians to intentionally scare the crap out of their overweight patients might yield good results, but it's an ethical no-go. A program that paid people twenty million dollars apiece to attain their ideal weight probably would achieve a nearly perfect success rate and prove once and for all that motivation is all it really takes for anyone to lose weight. But it's not feasible either. Nor can one simply muster a higher level of motivation to lose weight out of thin air. Maybe someday motivation will come in a pill. But for now it's really a matter of dumb luck—of stumbling upon just the right trigger at the right moment in one's life.

It's Not about the Food
Everyone has an overweight friend or acquaintance who says, "I've tried *everything* to lose weight. Nothing works for me!" These

frustrated men and women are prone to reject the idea that motivation is the true secret to weight loss because it seems to suggest that being overweight is their fault (whereas in fact it puts the blame on the biological, psychological, and social factors that make eating right and exercising seem so hard). It's more comfortable for those who haven't had their breakthrough yet to believe that the true secret to weight loss is yet to be discovered, or that their body is somehow immune to all diets—physically incapable of shedding excess fat. But there is no such thing as weight-loss immunity. Even the most frustrated serial dieter would lose a lot of weight if he was locked in a cage and forced to eat just 1,200 calories a day and walk three miles on a treadmill every morning—in other words, if his will was removed from the equation.

It's true that losing weight is harder for some people than it is for others. Scientists have identified specific genes that account for inter-individual differences in weight-loss ability. Interestingly, these genes affect the brain, rather than the body proper. People who struggle to lose weight often blame their lack of success on a "slow metabolism" (as Brandy Alles once did), but the real culprit is usually an inherent deficiency in self-control that is specific to eating. In extreme cases, such as the dreadful Prader-Willi syndrome, which is caused by overproduction of the hunger hormone ghrelin, eating restraint and healthy weight maintenance are impossible. But for the rest of us, an innate weakness in food-related impulse inhibition merely increases the amount of motivation that is required to lose weight. The secret is still the same and is still available; it's just more elusive.

In recent years, scientists have proposed that a sort of food addiction may hinder weight-loss efforts for many people. There is now strong evidence that high-fat and high-sugar diets alter brain function in some of the same ways that addictive narcotics do. The concept of food addiction remains controversial, but I believe in it for the most part because it is consistent with other evidence that being overweight is a matter of dependency on bad eating habits and not a matter of ignorance of how to lose weight. There is no medical cure for alcohol or drug addiction, yet people kick these habits every day. Like successful dieters, men and women who achieve sobriety do it in a hundred different ways—in groups or solo, abruptly or gradually, through religion or exercise, and so on. But behind these hundred ways there is always one thing: a cold determination not to fail this time. "All change is self-change," said the addiction psychologist James Prochaska.

Bariatric scientists have been slow to accept the fact that motivation is the real secret to weight loss, probably because there is so little they can do about it. But motivation has been winning more attention lately. A number of recent studies have shown that financial incentives to lose weight—incentives that are not accompanied by specific guidance on *how* to lose weight—yield at least as much weight loss as does specific guidance on how to lose weight delivered without incentives. But in all such cases the financial incentives have been small, hence weak.

Health insurers and other private enterprises have begun to use financial incentives to motivate weight loss in consumers and employees because they see that it can help their own bottom line. But until every man, woman, and child is given the opportunity to earn twenty million dollars by reaching a healthy weight, each of us is on his or her own to stumble upon the right motivation to lose weight. In the meantime, it can't hurt to recognize the invalidity of the idea that successful weight loss depends on eating a certain way.

The Myth of the Knowledge Barrier
One thing that all of the healthy-diet cults agree on is that nutritional knowledge is the key to attaining not just an ideal body weight, but also maximum health. They just disagree on the

knowledge itself. This makes it difficult to figure out which diet is based upon the truth. But knowledge is not really the key to slimness and health. The average ten-year-old knows enough about nutrition to transform her present way of eating into a healthy one. What she may lack, and may always lack, is the motivation to do it.

Knowledge itself can motivate, and the healthy-diet cults understand and exploit this fact, recruiting and retaining followers with a sacred doctrine that allows believers to bask in a feeling of group superiority. It works for some people sometimes. But for some of us, the diet-cult doctrines are too unbelievable to trigger a lasting dietary transformation. We need to find our motivation elsewhere.

6

It's a Bird! It's a Plane!
It's Superfood!

According to scripture, the Jewish people wandered homeless through the Sinai Desert for forty years after escaping captivity in Pharaoh's Egypt. According to Wikipedia, the Hebrew refugees finally settled in Canaan sometime around 1450 B.C.E., or possibly 1313 B.C.E. Their leader was Moses, who endured a great deal of kvetching from his hungry followers throughout those long forty years.

"If only we had died by the Lord's hand in Egypt!" they told him (Exodus 16:3). "There we sat around pots of meat and ate all the food we wanted, but you have brought us out into this desert to starve this entire assembly to death."

Moses was rescued from certain mutiny by the Lord Himself, who spoke soothing words to the prophet, promising to rain down a supernatural food from heaven during the night. Not above indulging in a bit of gloating, Moses trumpeted the good news among his grumbling brethren. Sure enough, when morning came a dew was upon the ground. The dew evaporated and left behind a dusting of thin flakes that were (says scripture) "white like coriander seed."

"What is it?" the people asked Moses.

"It is the bread the Lord has given you to eat," he said.

The Hebrew words for "What is it?" are *man hu*. An apocryphal theory posits that *man hu* eventually became *manna*.

In the Book of Exodus, which Moses is believed to have written by his own hand, manna is described as tasting "like wafers made with honey." It did not come in a ready-to-eat form. The Jews prepared the providential provender by grinding it with a hand mill or crushing it with a mortar and then either boiling it in a pot or shaping it into loaves for baking. Any manna left uneaten stank and was crawling with maggots by the next morning. This wasn't a problem, though, because a fresh supply of manna fell from heaven every night. Only on the night before the Sabbath did no manna fall.

God was proud of his manna and he commanded Moses to put some in a jar and save it to show to future generations. The gratitude of the people did not last, however. No sooner had they forgotten their hunger than they decided they were sick of eating nothing but manna all the time.

"If only we had meat to eat!" they complained. "We remember the fish we ate in Egypt at no cost—also the cucumbers, melons, leeks, onions, and garlic. But now we have lost our appetite; we never see anything but this manna!"

Not one to brook insubordination, God threatened to fill his people so full of the meat they craved that it came out of their nostrils. He later softened his position and brought a plague upon the people as they ate the meat he generously provided. After that it was back to manna. Chastened, the Jews held their tongues for the better part of the next forty years, but eventually their patience wore out and they grumbled anew.

"Why have you brought us up out of Egypt to die in the wilderness?" they cried, addressing God and Moses corporately. "There is no bread! There is no water! And we detest this miserable food!"

This time God sent poisonous snakes to attack his people. Many were killed. The survivors repented and went back to eating manna until, at long last, the Jews succeeded in sacking the city of Canaan (slaughtering every man, woman, and child therein) and claiming it as their new home. According to extra-biblical tradition, manna ceased to fall the very day Moses died.

Archeologists say that the Jews' forty years of desert wandering and the Exodus that preceded it and the captivity in Egypt that preceded that did not really happen, and that manna never existed. But if manna *did* exist, and if the Jews did eat it almost exclusively for forty years, then we know what was in it—or much of what was in it, anyway.

There are forty-six individual nutrients, including water (which isn't always counted as a nutrient), that are classified as essential to human life. If the wandering Jews got their water from the usual sources, then manna must have contained the other forty-five. There are fourteen essential vitamins: A, nine different B vitamins, C, D, E, and K. The body is able to synthesize vitamin D when exposed to sunlight, and the wandering Jews had more than enough of that, being without permanent shelter in the Sinai Desert, but I think it's safe to assume that God would have included vitamin D in manna just in case.

The number of essential minerals is seventeen. They are calcium, chloride, chromium, cobalt, copper, iodine, iron, magnesium, manganese, molybdenum, nickel, phosphorus, potassium, selenium, sodium, sulfur, and zinc. Some of these nutrients are referred to as trace minerals because they are needed in very small amounts. There is also an undefined number of so-called "ultra-trace" minerals—among them boron, silicon, and arsenic (yes, arsenic)—which are present in the human body in only the tiniest amounts, yet participate in critical metabolic functions and may also be essential for all we know. It seems very likely that manna (if it existed) contained any and all essential ultratrace minerals.

Then there are the nine essential amino acids: histidine, iso-leucine, leucine, lysine, methionine, phenylalanine, threonine, tryptophan, and valine. The body is able to make the other eleven amino acids that human life depends on from these nine, but it cannot make these nine from the other eleven, so we know that manna contained at least the nine essentials.

Finally, there are two essential fatty acids: alpha-linolenic acid and linoleic acid. Given an adequate supply of these two fats, the body can do without the dozens of other varieties of fats found in all animal foods and many plant foods. There is no doubt that manna (again, if there ever was such a thing) contained adequate amounts of the essential fatty acids.

By definition, a diet that provided all of the essential nutrients and only the essential nutrients would suffice to support basic health and to sustain life for a normal duration. But it is highly probable that a person placed on such a minimally adequate diet would have some complaints. For example, fiber is not an essential nutrient but the body's plumbing works much better with it. Similarly, there are no essential carbohydrates, but it's unlikely that a person would feel up to much activity—or even much thought—on a zero-carbohydrate diet.

Since it is reported that manna tasted like honey, we may specu-late that it did contain some carbohydrate, perhaps even sugars. I would wager that manna was packed with other goodies too. It's hard to imagine God would have gone to the trouble to create a miracle food that was barely sufficient. Even if it did provide only what was essential, however, manna qualified as a bona fide miracle food, and not only because it fell from the sky. There is not a single food found in nature that contains all of the nutrients that are essential to sustain human life.

From Miracle Foods to Superfoods

Real or not, manna wasn't the only food in the diet of the ancient Jewish people that was considered a gift from God. Bread was another. The importance of bread to the Jews of Moses' time cannot be overstated. It was their chief staple. When bread was abundant, the people flourished; when it was not, the people suffered.

The Israelites had their own special ways of making and using bread—for example, baking it without leavening for certain religious feasts—so that this food became even more important to their cultural identity than its utility alone justified. The specialness of bread was so completely accepted among the children of Abraham that the word "bread" was used as a synonym for food.

Wine too was viewed as a gift from the Lord to his chosen people, but of a different sort—not a staple like bread but a special treat that the Creator intended to "gladden the heart of man" and to "treat infirmities." Wine had a special role in celebrations and religious rituals, including divine offerings. It is no accident that Jesus asked his Jewish disciples to remember him in bits of bread and sips of wine. The way had been prepared.

The Jews of antiquity were not alone in recognizing a divine presence in select foods. Many ancient peoples believed that the foods they most depended on and most relished—and which therefore were most central to their cultural identity—were celestial gifts invested with supernatural qualities that made them fundamentally different from other foods. The potato (which is the subject of the next chapter) was quite literally worshipped by some ancient peoples of South America for whom it was a vital staple. Chocolate was known to these same peoples as "the food of the gods" because of the pleasure it conferred. (I'll have more to say about chocolate in Chapter 9.)

Anthropologists say that when cultures of the past saw God in certain foods they were essentially exaggerating the goodness of their most treasured foods. What's funny is how little has changed. Today many people still exaggerate the goodness of their most treasured foods, but they do so in a different way. Instead of calling them "foods of the gods," they call them *superfoods*.

The oldest recorded use of the word "superfood" is to be found in a poem published in a Jamaican newspaper during the First World War. The poet attached the neologism specifically to wine, in reference to the beverage's mood-altering effects. His thinking seems to have been that whereas foods merely sustain life, a superfood *enhances* life.

When used as a prefix, the word "super" may designate either a superior example of a particular type of thing or a phenomenon that transcends its type. Superman, for example, shares the essence of normal men but is superior to them. The supernatural, on the other hand, lies beyond the natural. The poet who coined the term "superfood" clearly had the "supernatural" sense of "super" in mind. A person cannot live by wine alone. Wine is an imitation of food that enriches life when one is already well nourished.

If manna was a superfood, it was so in a very different sense— namely, the Superman sense: a regular food, only better. This other meaning of the word "superfood" was the one assigned to it in its second-oldest recorded use. An article published in Alberta, Canada's *Lethbridge Herald* in 1949 referred to a certain muffin as "a superfood that contained all the known vitamins and some that had not been discovered." Now *that* sounds like something closer to manna—something a person could live on in a pinch.

So by the middle of the twentieth century, two distinct meanings of the word "superfood" were available. On the one hand, a superfood might be thought of as a sort of medicine, not sufficient on its own to sustain life but still valuable as a life-enhancing bonus for the well fed. Alternatively, a superfood might be defined as a source of complete basic nutrition. Both meanings remain with us today, but only one is in common use. If you had no clue which it was, you could find out very quickly by looking through one of the many popular books on superfoods.

David Wolfe's *Superfoods*, for example, identifies and describes the author's picks for "The Top 10 Superfoods." There are individual chapters on each of them: goji berries, cacao, maca, bee products (honey, bee pollen, royal jelly, and propolis), spirulina, AFA blue-green algae, marine phytoplankton, aloe vera, hempseed, and coconuts.

Goji berries (also known as wolfberries) are bright orange berries that come from a Chinese shrub. They were used in traditional Chinese medicine to promote longevity. They are full of exotic antioxidant phytonutrients and a few familiar vitamins. However, they lack some essential minerals as well as both of the essential fatty acids and more than one essential amino acid. One could not live on them.

Cacao beans are, of course, the source of chocolate. Like goji berries, they are chock full of nonessential phytonutrients with antioxidant properties. Eating them is believed to be good for the cardiovascular system. But again, like goji berries, cacao beans lack some essential nutrients, including vitamin C. If you tried to live on cacao beans, you might eventually die of scurvy.

Maca is a root plant native to Peru that has been used in folk medicine for centuries, primarily as an aphrodisiac. Although it contains a variety of essential and nonessential nutrients, maca is really more of a medicine than a food. One would never make a meal out of it, or even a snack. It must be powdered to be easily ingested.

Three of the four bee products—pollen, royal jelly, and propolis—are not properly foods either. Traditionally they were
consumed strictly as medicines, and today they are used only
as supplements. Honey is a food, of course, but one with a very
limited nutrition profile. Granted, John the Baptist is said to have
survived on nothing but locusts and honey. But of these two foods,
locusts probably did more to keep him breathing.

Spirulina is a type of microalgae. Its nutrient profile is impres-
sive. Spirulina is among the most protein-rich non-animal foods
in the world, and it contains goodly amounts of carbohydrate, fat,
and fiber, plus all the phytonutrients you would expect in a food
so luminously green. Yet even spirulina does not have everything.
Nutritiondata.com has given spirulina a "Completeness Score" of
sixty-nine on its 100-point scale of nutritional balance. Plain old
spinach has a Completeness Score of ninety-three.

AFA blue-green algae is virtually the same thing as spirulina except that it grows in only one place in the entire world:
Klamath Lake in Oregon. According to David Wolfe, AFA
blue-green algae contains more chlorophyll, more minerals,
more phycocyanin, more vitamin C, and more essential fatty
acids than spirulina. Why, then, did Wolfe bother to include its
inferior cousin spirulina among his Top 10 Superfoods? Because,
he wrote, "years of experience have demonstrated to me that
spirulina is more friendly to human metabolism and digestion
than AFA blue-green algae." I think that's a polite way of saying
that you can forget about trying to live on AFA blue-green algae
exclusively unless you don't mind diarrhea.

Marine phytoplankton is yet another tiny green sea ration. The
big difference between it and spirulina and AFA blue-green algae
is that marine phytoplankton is a plant, not a bacterium. Some
species of whale thrive on a plankton-based diet. Humans could
too if we had baleens—mouth filters that sieve huge amounts of
plankton out of seawater—but we don't.

Aloe vera is a cactus-like plant native to the Mediterranean whose distinctive sap has been used medicinally since antiquity. Aloe sap has two components: gel and latex. There is evidence that topical application of the gel to the skin accelerates wound healing. Ingestion of the latex is an effective treatment for constipation. Unfortunately, it is also carcinogenic. For this reason the aloe juices that are sold for drinking are made from the gel, not the latex. But there are no substantiated health benefits associated with consuming aloe gel, and in any case aloe gel is not especially nourishing because it contains no carbohydrate, fat, or protein. One would quickly starve to death on an all-aloe diet.

Hemp seeds are (need I say?) the seeds of marijuana plants. As any pot smoker will tell you, hemp seeds won't get you high; however, they are rich in essential nutrients, including all nine essential amino acids and both essential fatty acids. Hulled hemp seeds are sold by the bag as a nutritious addition to baked goods, salads, oatmeal, and breakfast cereals. They're perfect for such uses, but they wouldn't make a good substitute for those other foods. Lacking vitamins A and C and calcium, hemp seeds are no manna.

Coconuts are used for flavoring more than they are for nutriment, but according to David Wolfe the Sanskrit word for the coconut palm is *kalpa vriksha*, which means, "the tree that supplies all that is needed to live." If this description were accurate, then coconuts would be a superfood in the Superman (and manna) sense. But in fact the coconut palm does not supply all that is needed for life. Coconut flesh lacks four essential vitamins and contains only trace amounts of a few others. Its Completeness Score is a paltry twenty-six.

David Wolfe explicitly defined superfoods in his book as "both a food and a medicine." But it's clear from his Top 10 list that Wolfe really thinks of superfoods as *foods that are used like medicines*—that is, in small doses that serve only to supplement the *mere* foods we actually fill our bellies with. Very much like wine, actually.

Other superfood evangelists define the class more broadly than David Wolfe does and their lists of top superfoods are therefore longer. But even these longer lists are generally skewed toward wine-type superfoods rather than manna-type superfoods. One of the most inclusive lists of superfoods is the one that Deborah Klein put in her book, *The 200 Superfoods That Will Save Your Life*. If I were given this list having no prior exposure to the concept of superfoods, my best guess would be that superfoods were nothing more than foods that were popularly regarded as "healthy" by health-conscious eaters.

There are many familiar, even mundane foods on Klein's list, some of which undoubtedly are eaten on occasion by the *least* health-conscious eaters. Popcorn is represented, as are maple syrup, cheese, and oatmeal. Klein makes a good case for the "superness" of each food in her catalog. The list is so inclusive, however, that one can't help but wonder about some of the foods left off it. Almond butter is among Klein's 200, but old-fashioned peanut butter is not. Red wine made the cut but white wine came up short. Black beans will save your life, according to Klein, but black-eyed peas, we are left to assume, will not.

It would take some effort, but you could construct a perfectly healthy diet that completely avoided all 200 of Deborah Klein's life-saving superfoods. It might be a little heavy on fava beans, macadamia nuts, bison, winter squash, sauropus (a green, leafy vegetable from Asia), dragon fruit, and beer, but Klein would have a hard time arguing that the diet was less nutritious than a diet constructed entirely from foods that were on her list.

If we accept that each of Deborah Klein's 200 life-saving superfoods is legitimately super in some way, then it becomes almost impossible to exclude *any* food that nature produces. Can we honestly say that even a single natural species that humans have chosen to incorporate into their diet is not super in some way? It seems to me that the only truly *non*-super foods are some of those that are heavily processed from natural sources, such as donuts. Under scrutiny, the concept of superfood becomes almost meaningless.

David Wolfe and Deborah Klein and other superfood advocates cite science to validate their choices. When allowed to speak for itself, though, science does not support the separation of foods into the categories of mere foods and superfoods. Yet people persist in doing it anyway, and for much the same reason that ancient cultures attributed supernatural qualities to their favorite foods. So uniquely important is food in human identity formation that there exists within each of us an impulse to exaggerate the goodness of the foods we most identify with. Far from having eradicated this impulse, science has only helped us disguise it.

Selling Superfoods

These days, superfoods are quite popular among vegetarians, vegans, raw-foodists, environmentalists, and organic eaters. But nowhere are superfoods more exalted than in the subculture of multi-level marketing, that shadowy industry in which each company's customer base and sales force are made up of the same people. I'm talking about Amway, Mary Kay, and other outfits whose "independent representatives" recruit new independent representatives, who do the same, ad infinitum. Like Ponzi schemes, MLM's are organized as pyramids. Independent reps get a cut of the product sales made by all of the reps underneath them in their network. The difference is that there are no products in a Ponzi scheme—money is just shuffled upward from the base to the top of the pyramid. MLM's are legally required to sell products to distinguish themselves from Ponzi schemes (which are not legal), but these products are sold with a wink and a nod.

Everyone knows it's all about signing up new reps. That's how the real money is made. If you are invited to an Amway meeting or a Mary Kay party you will hear a little talk about skincare products or makeup and a lot more talk about the opportunity to get rich quick as your own boss. Only a tiny fraction of MLM products are sold to individuals who are not themselves independent representatives selling the same products.

The specific types of products that work best in this industry are cheap consumables that tend to be purchased frequently. The ideal multilevel marketing products are those whose cheapness is easily disguised, so they can be sold at big markups. Superfoods—or certain kinds of superfoods, anyway—fit this description perfectly. The superfoods that MLM's sell are not the fresh, perishable herbs and fruits that are available at reasonable prices at any supermarket. Instead, they are *engineered* superfoods: bottled juices of exotic fruits and canisters containing special mixtures of powdered plant extracts that are hyped as being even healthier than nature's bounty in its natural state.

The association of multi-level marketing with processed superfoods goes right back to the beginning. The first modern nutritional supplement and the first multi-level marketing company were created by the same man. Dr. Carl Rehnborg developed the multivitamin in the 1930s. The company he founded to sell this product and a few others, called Nutrilite, started with a traditional business model but in 1945 switched over to a direct-selling model, where virtually every customer also sold the products. Nutrilite was later bought by Amway, the world's largest MLM, with almost twelve billion dollars in total sales in 2013.

The most successful MLM of this century is MonaVie, a Mormon-affiliated company that sells superfood juices made from açai fruit, which is among Deborah Klein's 200 superfoods that will save our lives and is also among ten "Honorable Mentions" in David Wolfe's much more exclusive ranking of the top superfoods. In 2008, *Newsweek* writer Tony Dokoupil attended a MonaVie rally led by company cofounder Dallin Larsen. Here's how he described it:

> Flanked by a Ferrari, a Maserati, a Bentley, a Rolls-Royce and a Lamborghini, Dallin Larsen paced the stage, swigging deeply from a bottle in his hand. "I'll tell you what," said the tanned 49-year-old, opening his arms to the 4,000-person crowd, people are "looking for something they can count on, they can depend on, that's constant." The stirring scene would not be out of place at a megachurch revival—except Larsen's event, organized this June in Orlando, Fla., was bent on earning sales rather than salvation. The object of hope was not God but a dark purple fruit juice called MonaVie.

Multi-level marketing businesses are often likened to cults because their culture is overtly religious, their leaders often wield outsized influence over the lives of members, and their disaffected members often have a hard time getting out. Sociologists have observed that the cult-like culture of multi-level marketing is critical to the industry's survival. The greatest challenge to the viability of the multi-level marketing industry is the fact that the business opportunities it offers are *extremely bad opportunities* for people whose goal is to get rich quick while working from home. It is estimated that more than ninety-nine out of one hundred independent representatives in any given MLM lose money, and more than half either quit or become inactive within a year of signing up. And the industry has now been around long enough that its awful track record is no secret. Everyone knows that there are ninety-nine losers for every winner. No person who is thinking rationally would ever fall for an MLM pitch. To successfully recruit new reps, MLM's must manipulate recruits into making an irrational decision to sign up.

MLM rallies like the one Tony Dokoupil attended are therefore carefully orchestrated to paralyze the reasoning faculties of attendees. A charismatic leader is introduced with hyperbolic praise and held under a spotlight, his voice amplified to coax out the audience's readiness to worship; powerful symbols of luxury are used to inflame greed; stirring music foments an emotionally charged altered state; an appealing quasi-religious doctrine— whose core precept, first articulated in Napoleon Hill's *Think and Grow Rich* (the "MLM bible"), is that wanting things makes them come to you—is preached; and the amazing brainwashing power of large groups is unleashed to finish the job.

These social tools of manipulation are the most tried-and-true means that multi-level marketing companies use to place new recruits in an irrational mindset when they make a decision about whether to sign up. But the most successful companies, like MonaVie, exploit an additional tool: superfoods.

Earlier I noted that the ideal MLM product is a cheap consumable that is easily sold at a premium, like engineered superfoods. But even better is a product of this sort that new recruits can be convinced is *supernatural*. Clothes, cosmetics, and electronics don't have that power. Only foods have the potential to be seen as gifts from God (perhaps not literally in this modern age of science but effectively, at least). In its greedy canniness the multilevel marketing industry has recognized that the ancient human inclination to designate certain special foods as miraculous is still with us, albeit cloaked in science lately. This is not a rational disposition. So when MLM's sell engineered superfoods, they no longer have to work so hard to convince new recruits that a business opportunity that ends disastrously for 99 percent will work out great for them. They just have to convince them that joining a community of people who drink forty-dollar bottles of exotic miracle juices will bring them contentment and eternal health, which is much easier.

Multi-level marketing companies promote their engineered superfoods in a far more over-the-top way than folks like David Wolfe and Deborah Klein promote nature's superfoods. If you've ever been recruited by an independent representative for a superfood-selling MLM, it has been suggested to you that you cannot achieve complete health without using the product being peddled. Do not ask why nature allowed human beings to exist in conditions that did not permit perfect health until this product was invented. Ask only this: "Do I want perfect health or not?"

While all MLM superfoods are supplements rather than staples, their marketing always positions them as essential in the way of manna. One is made to understand that the cost of refusing them is something just short of a divine plague of snakes. Indeed, one of the more successful superfood-selling MLM's (and one of the more notorious, having been sued for fraud) is called Mannatech.

A typical multilevel marketing superfood is Healose, which its maker, a smaller MLM called NutriHarmony, describes as "one of the most powerful health products ever created." The active ingredient in Healose is fulvic acid, which is an organic acid derived from humus, a variety of dirt, not to be confused with hummus, made from garbanzo beans. NutriHarmony's website states that "Hundreds of advanced studies coming from scientists all around the world proclaim the benefits of Fulvic Acid to be 'incredible', 'amazing', 'miraculous', 'magical', 'phenomenal'! Research shows that Fulvic Acid has actual fountain-of-youth-like health properties."

A quick search through the U.S. National Library of Medicine's PubMed online database—which contains abstracts of every study published in a major English-language peer-reviewed medical journal since 1966—exposes these statements as utterly baseless. Of the twenty-two million studies available on PubMed at the time I conducted my search, exactly *five* concerned the effects of fulvic acid on human health. The most mind-blowing of these studies reported that fulvic acid was a fairly effective treatment for eczema—when applied topically.

If Healose is no more nourishing than the dirt it comes from, other MLM superfood products are actually beneficial. MonaVie seems pretty healthy to me. Indeed, a study published in the respected *Nutrition Journal* reported that one month of açai supplementation reduced fasting glucose and insulin levels as well as total cholesterol in overweight adults. That's nice, but thirty days of eating spinach salads probably would have produced similar effects.

MonaVie has run afoul of the U.S. Food and Drug Administration for making benefit claims that go far beyond reduced fasting glucose levels in the overweight. The company's official messaging has since been reined in, but its independent representatives continue to credit the juice for astonishing health miracles when recruiting their friends and neighbors to join—a problem the company is aware of but, alas, powerless to control. In any case, as good as açai juice may be for the body, plain old orange juice is probably just as good at a tenth of the cost.

The Myth of Extraordinary Foods
Most healthy-diet cults keep lists of favorite foods. These lists are highly disparate. The Mediterranean diet fetishizes olive oil. The Paleo Diet venerates meat. Some of the diet cults of the late nineteenth century singled out milk as nature's "perfect food." Despite these differences, the many diet cults share a tendency to exaggerate the goodness of the foods they like best, either stating outright or implying that these foods are drastically healthier than other foods. Not every diet cult talks of superfoods, but each encourages some degree of worship of its special foods. This phenomenon is a legacy from ancient times, when different

cultures thought of their most treasured foods as supernatural gifts of divine origin.

The multi-level marketing industry capitalizes on our weakness for miracle foods to gain dishonest profits. Yet there is something dishonest about any effort to promote particular superfoods that enlists science in support of its boosterism. A fair interpretation of the relevant science says that there is no God in any food. Either that, or there is a little God in almost every food.

7

Consider the Potato

Robert Atkins was no friend of the potato. He made this perfectly clear when he was interviewed by CNN's Larry King on January 6, 2003, at the height of the low-carb diet craze for which Atkins was largely responsible. During the interview, King appeared to have trouble wrapping his head around the idea that Atkins ate all of the high-fat foods (such as hamburger patties with cheese) he wanted, but steered clear of low-fat foods containing carbohydrate (such as hamburger buns).

"So, in other words, you have the steak but you don't have the bread," King said dubiously.

"And you don't have the potatoes either, for that matter," Atkins rejoined.

"What's an Atkins dinner?" King asked later in the conversation.

"Well, now you're talking about my wife, who is such a great cook," Atkins said, perhaps conscious of his wife's eyes watching him on a monitor in the nearby green room or on a TV screen back home.

"She'll cook?" King asked, seeming to mean "Wait—she's actually willing to cook *your* way?"

"She has incredible fish, incredible fowl, and all kinds of meat—rack of lamb, lamb chops," Atkins gushed.

"Eat the fatty part of the lamb chop too?" King challenged.

"Yes, I eat that," Atkins said, a bit hesitantly. "And just with a lot of vegetables."

"Any potatoes?" King deadpanned.

"No, not the potatoes, but an awful lot—"

"How about a sweet potato?" King interrupted.

"Rarely," Atkins said flatly.

Anyone watching this interview who was among the fourteen million purchasers of *Dr. Atkins' New Diet Revolution* would have known already how Atkins felt about the humble spud. The word "potato" appears thirty-two times in history's best-selling diet book. The general flavor of these references is conveyed by a line on page 254: "Baked stuffed potatoes are an absolute no-no."

In another part of the book, Atkins pointed out that the problem with potatoes was that they were too *starchy*. He was discussing the glycemic index, a scientific scale that scores individual foods according to their immediate effect on the blood glucose level. The greater the glucose spike, Atkins explained, the higher the food's GI score—and high was bad. He then drew the reader's attention to a boxed table that listed a number of familiar foods in descending order of their glycemic index scores. The baked potato was near the top with a score of eighty-five.

"It's interesting to browse through the list," Atkins observed. "Notice that the baked potato ranks exceptionally high. Starch converts to glucose in the bloodstream with great rapidity."

Atkins believed that high blood glucose levels were bad because they stimulated the release of insulin, a hormone that aids in the conversion of glucose to body fat. He recommended eating in a way that kept blood glucose levels low, forcing the body to use stored fat to keep itself functioning and thereby promoting weight loss. Avoiding potatoes and other starchy foods was one of the most effective ways to keep the blood glucose level low, Atkins said.

In 2003, one in six Americans was on some version of the Atkins Nutritional Approach, as it was officially known. So popular was this anti-potato diet that it had a measurable effect on the potato market—and Atkins wasn't sorry about it.

"When eating in a restaurant, ask your server to replace your rice or potato with a serving of vegetables," he advised.

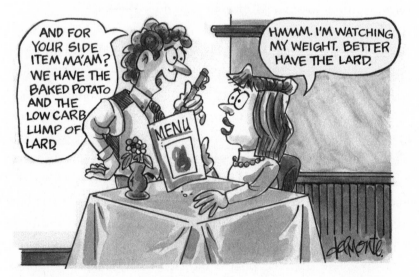

Millions of Americans did just that. Restaurants adapted. At the climax of the trend, thousands of restaurants offered low-carb menu items that removed potatoes from their traditional places. Meat and potatoes became meat and . . . *something else.* Even the unlikeliest chains, among them Ruth's Chris Steak House, hopped on the bandwagon with special low-carb offerings such as a sixteen-ounce rib-eye with a side of spinach.

Low-carb dieters also bought fewer fresh potatoes for consumption at home. While potatoes remained the most popular vegetable in the American diet, sales dropped markedly in the period of Atkins's reign. Overall potato consumption declined by ten pounds per person annually in the United States from its pre-Atkins peak. An 8 percent drop in demand for potatoes caused prices to dip and potato stockpiles to swell. Growers had little choice but to reduce production, which decreased by 7 percent in the Atkins heyday. Potato stocks in the thirteen major potato-growing states decreased by a similar amount.

The fallout spread far beyond the borders of the nation where it all started. Potato sales in Scotland, for example, plummeted 10 percent between 2003 and 2004. The following year, potato sales began a downward slide in Ireland—Ireland!

The industry tried to fight back. In 2004, the United States Potato Board launched a four-million-dollar "Healthy Potato" campaign to rehabilitate the maligned tuber's reputation. New product labels were created to draw attention to the nutritional virtues of the vegetable—low calorie density, high vitamin C concentration, loads of zinc. Advertisements bearing the same message were placed in newspapers and popular magazines. The potato growers also hired nutritionists to attack the principles of the Atkins diet and undermine the credibility of the man behind it. These efforts were undercut by the potato industry itself when it unveiled an ill-conceived hedge: a genetically modified "low-carb" potato.

It's possible that the potato industry's vilification of Robert Atkins was a bit out of proportion to Atkins's actual level of disdain for the potato. While Atkins did preach general potato avoidance, he stopped short of lumping potatoes together with soft drinks and Skittles. As bad as starch was in Atkins's mind, sugar was worse. Sugary foods and drinks, whose glycemic index scores were the highest in the food kingdom, had no place whatsoever in the Atkins program, whereas potatoes were permitted in small amounts under special circumstances. Only dieters who had already reached their weight-loss goal were eligible for this indulgence. But goal attainment alone was not enough. The successful dieter also had to demonstrate what Atkins termed a "low level of metabolic resistance," by which he meant a low propensity to regain weight in response to a little dietary laxity. If both of these conditions were met, Atkins allowed the dieter to eat as many as fifty or sixty grams of carbohydrate per day, or about the amount of carbohydrate in a bowl of oatmeal with milk and banana slices (make it last!).

"If you're careful," Atkins promised, "and you find you don't go into a weight-gaining spiral, you may be able to have even an occasional potato and some wild rice."

Clearly, Atkins would not have dangled this hope if he believed that potatoes were truly deadly. But such nuances were lost on most Atkins dieters, who decided that what he had really meant to say was that potatoes were indeed deadly and should never be eaten. So they did not eat them. Even the low-carb potato flopped.

A Propitious Esculent

The potato is native to Central America, originating some forty million years ago in the areas now known as Guatemala and Mexico and then migrating southward to the harsh, high elevations of the Andes mountains, where it grew especially well. Today's big, white, smooth russet scarcely resembles its wild antecedents. Nor did these antecedents much resemble each other. Hundreds of species of potato existed in the rarefied, equatorial habitat that suited them best before human cultivation homogenized them. They came in a rainbow of colors, and most were small and gnarled in shape.

The edible tuber is only one part of the potato plant. The above-ground parts include stalks, leaves, and rather pretty flowers. The below-ground tuber is actually a section of the stem grown fat as a source of stored energy for the rest of the plant and is the main reason the potato plant is able to thrive in challenging environments through seasons of bitter cold and scarce water. Few plants stash away high-energy starch for use in hard times quite like the potato.

The engorged section of stem that we know as the potato proper serves a second function besides that of supplying reserve energy. The so-called "eyes" of the potato produce buds that eventually become new potato plants. Another special characteristic of the potato is that it can reproduce in two ways. In addition to cloning itself underground, the potato reproduces sexually above ground through the pollination of seeds that are produced by the plant's flowers.

Humans did not exist in Central and South America until they arrived from Siberia by way of North America between 16,000 and 14,000 years ago at the tail end of the Journey of Man. Archaeological evidence suggests that humans began to eat and even cultivate potatoes very soon after discovering them. In 1976 the remarkably well-preserved remains of an ancient camp were discovered at a place called Monte Verde in southern Chile. Among the items found there were cooked potatoes. The site was dated to approximately 10,500 B.C.E., marking it as the oldest known place of human occupancy in the New World.

Scientists consider it a great mystery that humans began to eat potatoes so soon after first encountering them. Most wild potatoes have a bitter taste and contain high levels of toxic compounds called glycoalkaloids. Yet people ate them anyway. You can't ask for a more powerful illustration of the level of dietary adaptation that was required of our ancestors—and which they proved capable of—as they peopled the earth.

The potato offered its first samplers a number of virtues to compensate for its shortcomings. The greatest of these was its rich carbohydrate content. Carbs are to animals what super-high-octane gasoline is to automobiles. They are nature's best source of fast energy for activity, and as such they were a critical component of the diets of all ancient peoples. Before they started eating potatoes, the nomadic first Central and South Americans would have gotten most of their carbs from native fruits such as papayas and tomatoes. The problem with such fruits is that they are seasonal and therefore unavailable during much of the year. Potatoes are seasonal too, but unlike fruits and other edible plants they can be stored or even left underground for months before they spoil. Potatoes presented to their original human eaters a uniquely reliable year-round source of precious carbohydrate.

A potato contains twice as much carbohydrate as a tomato, but that's not all it has going for it nutritionally. Potatoes contain a small amount of high-quality protein with a higher concentration of essential amino acids than whey protein (a favorite among bodybuilders) and a higher "biological value" than soy protein. The potato is also, as previously mentioned, rich in vitamin C and zinc, as well as in B vitamins, potassium, fiber (in the skin) and even antioxidants.

Human beings can live indefinitely on a diet in which potatoes are the sole source of food energy. This was first demonstrated scientifically by the Danish physician and nutritionist Mikkel Hindhede in the late nineteenth century. To test the hypothesis that potatoes might be used to stave off famine in times of national crisis, Hindhede lived off potatoes and potato water plus small amounts of milk and butter for several months. Far from suffering any negative health effects on this limited diet, Hindhede came away from it having concluded that "man can retain full vigor for a year or longer on a diet of potatoes and fat."

A decade later, a pair of Polish researchers, Stanislaw Kon and Aniela Klein, attempted to confirm Hindhede's findings. They placed themselves on an all-potato diet (supplemented with a bit of coffee and fruit) for 167 days. In a paper that summarized the results of this trial Kon and Klein blandly remarked, "The digestion was excellent throughout the experiment and both subjects felt very well." Kon even managed to keep up a vigorous athletic training regimen during the experiment.

The potato was first domesticated in what is now Peru roughly eight thousand years ago. It did not happen all at once. The process was stepwise, perhaps largely accidental. Gatherers first selected the best-tasting and least poisonous potatoes from wild patches. They then discovered that if they left some of the better potato plants in the ground, the next crop was better still. Finally they began planting favored varieties of potato in managed fields.

Advances in cooking methods were as important as innovations in farming techniques in establishing the potato as a staple for the earliest South Americans. It was discovered that mixing potatoes with a bit of a certain kind of clay before eating them prevented the stomach pains caused by those pesky glycoalkaloids. Later the same people created *chuño*, a sort of freeze-dried potato cake that was free of toxins and stored well.

The first potato growers living around Lake Titicaca could not have known that the food they had domesticated would remain the most calorically productive crop on earth for more than 10,000 years. To this day the potato yields more food energy per planted acre than any other thing planted. The first potato growers knew nothing about calories, but they were well able to appreciate what their chief staple did for them. The abundance that flowed from potato cultivation made possible the first great South American civilization, that of the Moche, which thrived between 0 and 600 B.C.E. and whose surviving artifacts suggest a degree of potato worship. The Moche gave way to the Tiwanaku, a more highly developed civilization based even more squarely on potato cultivation. After several hundred years on top, the Tiwanaku were supplanted by the Inca, the first and last true empire of South America, for whom the potato was one of two core staples. (The other was maize.)

The Inca met a premature demise when Francisco Pizarro's party of Spanish adventurers landed near the city of Cuzco in 1532 and immediately started shooting. The potato was one of many New World curiosities that reached Europe soon afterward, but more than two and a half centuries would pass before Europeans recognized that the potato could advance the security and health of their societies no less than it had in the Pre-Columbian societies of South America. The reason it took so long was that the potato was judged unattractive, dirty, and bland in comparison to other New World foods such as the tomato, which gained popularity in Europe more quickly. The spud's popularity was not helped by a superstitious belief that eating potatoes caused leprosy.

It was war that ultimately motivated Europe to give the potato a second look and a first real chance on a broad scale. Wars ravaged the continent throughout the seventeenth and eighteenth centuries. There were more civilians killed by famine in these conflicts than there were soldiers killed by bullets. Whether defending their own lands or invading foreign ones, troops routinely requisitioned, commandeered, destroyed, and trammeled grain crops, leaving nothing behind. Armies were less inclined to dig up fields of potatoes than to raid or burn a wheat-packed barn, however, and an infantry could march over a potato field without harming a single tuber. New potato farmers quickly recognized that, even in times of peace, potatoes offered a number of advantages compared to wheat and other grains, yielding many times more calories per planted acre and surviving frost and drought conditions that caused grain crops to fail. Initially resorted to in desperation, potatoes became first a subsistence food and then a commercial food of choice throughout Europe in the eighteenth century.

The potato's superiority to previous staple foods in Europe and elsewhere has been quantified. Historians have shown that population growth followed the advent of widespread potato farming everywhere from Switzerland to China. What's more, people not only grew in numbers after the potato arrived in these places, but they also grew measurably taller. It is no exaggeration to say that potatoes singlehandedly made almost the entire human race healthier than it had ever been.

Nowhere did the potato have a greater effect than in Ireland. The Irish took to the potato earlier and more unreservedly than any other European people because they were particularly desperate for food and the potato grew especially well on the Emerald Isle, unlike wheat, which prefers a drier climate. By the late seventeenth century, the potato was the chief source of calories in the Irish diet. Over the next century the population of the country doubled, and in the next fifty years it nearly doubled again despite high levels of emigration.

By the second quarter of the nineteenth century, one in three Irish lived on a virtually all-potato diet. Then the famine hit. Unlike famines associated with the failure of grain harvests, the Irish potato famine of 1845 to 1852 was caused not by drought but rather by a fungus that wiped out crops. One million people died in the famine and another million Irish emigrated to escape it.

Imagine a starving Irishman receiving a visit from a time traveler during this terrible crisis and being told that 150 years later, an American diet guru would condemn the potato as unhealthy and encourage people to abstain from eating potatoes, no matter how plentiful they might be. The inconceivable folly of this future might well have finished the poor fellow off.

When Carbs Went Bad

The great epiphany of Robert Atkins's life occurred in October 1963, when he read an article titled "A New Concept in the Treatment of Obesity" in the *Journal of the American Medical Association*. The article focused on the work of Alfred Pennington, a physician working for the DuPont chemical company who had a longstanding research interest in the treatment of obesity. Pennington had arrived at the conclusion that excess consumption of carbohydrate—particularly sugar—was the major cause of the rising rate of obesity in the United States. Naturally, this idea led him to believe that carbohydrate restriction was the most effective way to treat obesity. Pennington's hypothesis flew in the face of the dominant theory that obesity was caused by excessive fat intake and was best treated with a low-fat diet.

Atkins was intrigued by the carbohydrate hypothesis. At the time, he was a thirty-three-year-old physician with a private practice in Manhattan. He was also fat. So he placed himself on a low-carbohydrate diet and got good results. He then began to use the program on his overweight patients, who experienced similar success. Convinced that he was really on to something, Atkins threw himself into an effort to promote the low-carb philosophy to the multitudes. An appearance on the *Tonight Show* in 1965 led to an article in *Vogue* in 1970, which led to the publication of his first book in 1972. An updated version of the book released twenty years later was even more successful and gave Atkins a springboard from which to launch Atkins Nutritionals, a company that produced a full line of low-carb packaged foods and supplements.

Despite its unprecedented popularity, the Atkins diet never seemed like the sort of thing that was going to last forever. It had all the hallmarks of the fad diets that had come and gone before it—the Grapefruit Diet's extremism, the Slimfast Diet's hucksterism, and the Scarsdale Diet's guru factor. The inevitable wilting of the flower was just beginning when Atkins died from injuries sustained in a fall outside his Manhattan home in the spring of 2003, only a few weeks after his appearance on *Larry King Live*. Days later, the *Wall Street Journal* reported that Atkins had weighed 258 pounds at the time of his passing. Atkins's representatives did not dispute the number but claimed that it was the result of more than sixty pounds of weight gain caused by fluid retention while Atkins lay in a coma.

Even if the Atkins Nutritional Approach did not work especially well for its creator, it worked for plenty of other people. The first major scientific vindication of the Atkins diet was published a month after his death. A few dozen obese men and women were given copies of *Dr. Atkins' New Diet Revolution* with instructions to follow the diet plan it described. After six months they had lost an average of 15.2 pounds. Members of a control group that had been instructed to eat less and obey the government's Food Guide Pyramid lost only 6.9 pounds.

Subsequent long-term studies, however, poured cold water on the Atkins victory party. One such study was published in the *New England Journal of Medicine* in 2009. Researchers at the Harvard School of Public Health placed several hundred overweight men and women on four separate diets with vastly different ratios of macronutrients. The contribution of carbohydrate to total calories ranged from 35 percent to 65 percent. After six months, members of all four groups had lost the same amount of weight. After another eighteen months, members of all four groups had regained about a third of that weight.

Although the Atkins diet per se was not included in this comparison, the results challenged the notion that manipulating the amount of carbohydrate in the diet was the key to successful weight loss. If Robert Atkins's claim that excessive carbohydrate intake was the primary cause of obesity was correct, then a low-carb diet should have yielded more weight loss than low-fat and low-protein diets, but it did not.

Atkins himself defended the notion that carbs had made America fat by pointing out that a slight increase in the amount of carbohydrate consumed by the average American had occurred at about the same time the obesity crisis had started. But correlation is not causation. People get more colds when the weather is cold, but this doesn't mean that frosty air causes upper respiratory tract infections. A more convincing proof that eating lots of carbs makes people fat would be a general population study comparing carb intake with body weight and finding that people who eat a lot of carbs are heavier than people who eat relatively few carbs. A handful of large-scale observational studies have indeed looked at the relationship between individual carbohydrate intake levels and body weight. Most of them have found no influence of one on the other. The rest have found that people who eat the *most* carbs tend to weigh slightly *less* than those who eat the least.

The public figured out on its own that low-carb diets didn't work any better than the many fad diets that came along before it. Atkins Nutritionals shut its doors in 2005, a victim of waning interest in low-carb diets and of declining equity in the Atkins name. Even when the company was raking in 100 million dollars a year, it was difficult for some people to believe that a low-carb Atkins Endulge Chocolate Bar was healthier than a high-carb baked potato or a fructose-filled tangerine. Within a year of Atkins's passing, America was wholly wrapped up in the next fad: the South Beach Diet. But the South Beach Diet wasn't really new. It was just a revision of the Atkins diet. Its creator, cardiologist Arthur Agatston, followed Atkins's lead in blaming carbohydrate for making people fat. The difference was that Agatston drew a distinction between "good carbs" and "bad carbs," and said that only bad carbs made people fat.

The success of the South Beach Diet was the first indication that, despite the collapse of the dietary empire that bore his name, Robert Atkins would cast a very long shadow. Many if not most of the major diet trends of the past decade have been influenced by him. Would the gluten-free diet trend or the Paleo Diet have caught fire as each of them has if Atkins had not first changed the average eater's view of grains from healthy to unhealthy? Even in my little world, the realm of endurance sports, where carbohydrate was once king, the ripple effects of the Atkins doctrine have been felt. Many cyclists, runners, and triathletes now train and eat to become "fat adaptive" and to reduce their dependence on carbohydrate as a muscle fuel. This they do despite the fact that the diet of the world's best endurance athletes, the runners of East Africa, is more than 75 percent carbohydrate.

And Then There's the Potato

In 1995, Susanna Holt, a biochemist at the University of Sydney, Australia, designed an experiment whose purpose was to compare the effects of different foods on short-term satiety and appetite. She selected thirty-eight foods and prepared 240-calorie portions of each. The specific foods were as follows: baked beans, beef, boiled potatoes, apple, banana, brown rice, cake, cheese, croissant, cookies, crackers, donut, eggs, french fries, "grain" bread, grapes, ice cream, jellybeans, lentils, ling fish, Mars Bar, orange, pasta, peanuts, popcorn, potato chips, white bread, white rice, "wholemeal" bread, whole-wheat pasta, yogurt, and seven kinds of breakfast cereal.

Because of differences in calorie density, the amounts of the various foods that were needed to supply 240 calories varied greatly. Just two ounces of donut supplied 240 calories, for example, compared to twelve ounces of grapes.

Holt recruited thirteen volunteers and asked them to eat a single, 240-calorie portion of each of the thirty-eight foods on separate occasions. After consuming each food, the volunteers were asked to rate their hunger level every fifteen minutes for two hours. At that point, the volunteers were led to a buffet, where they were instructed to eat as much (or as little) of a standardized meal as they desired. Holt counted the number of calories the subjects ate in these meals and combined this data with the subjects' hunger ratings to create a "satiety index" for each food.

Like the glycemic index, Holt's satiety index used white bread as a reference food and assigned it a score of 100. Of the thirty-eight foods compared in the study, none scored lower than croissants. Two hours after eating croissants, the subjects felt hungrier and ate more than they did after eating any other food. The croissant's satiety index score was a pitiful forty-seven.

The highest satiety index score, by a vast margin, was achieved by—you guessed it—boiled potatoes. The satiety index score of boiled potatoes was 323. The second-highest score was 225, which went to ling fish. No other food came close to filling up the volunteers or reducing their subsequent meal size as much as boiled potatoes did.

One of the reasons boiled potatoes are so filling is that potatoes have a low calorie density. The volunteers in Holt's study had to eat ten ounces of the stuff to get 240 calories. Interestingly, the two other forms of potatoes included in the study—fries and chips—earned much lower satiety index scores. Fries came in at 116 and chips at ninety-one. Frying in oil makes these foods much more calorie dense and thus also much less satisfying, calorie for calorie, than potatoes cooked in other ways.

One would expect foods with stronger short-term satiety effects to have beneficial long-term effects on body weight. In other words, one would expect people who ate a lot of croissants to be fatter than people who ate a lot of boiled potatoes. Recent studies have generally confirmed that the short-term effects of individual foods on satiety do correlate with long-term effects of the same foods on body weight. The problem for potatoes, however, is that they are consumed mostly in fried forms these days, and according to at least one study *fried* potatoes cause more long-term weight gain than any other food. While it is clearly frying rather than the potato itself that is to blame, the typical health-conscious eater today blames the potato, particularly its starch content. The bad reputation that was wrongly bestowed upon the potato by Robert Atkins persists despite continuing scientific buttressing of its goodness, including one analysis which determined that white potatoes offer more total nutritional value per unit cost than any other food except their cousin the sweet potato.

In 2011, the United States Department of Agriculture introduced a proposal to improve the quality of school lunches by limiting the amount of "starchy vegetables"—potatoes, corn, green peas, and lima beans—that could be served to schoolchildren. The potato industry fought vigorously against the ham-handed proposal. The head of the Washington State Potato Commission, Chris Voigt, was so personally exasperated by the stupidity of the government's bid to take *vegetables* rather than fried oils out of the mouths of youngsters that he publicly vowed to defend the potato's healthfulness by eating nothing but potatoes—twenty spuds a day without toppings—for sixty straight days.

If Robert Atkins had been available to counsel Voigt, he would have warned the zealous potato advocate that two months on an almost pure-carb diet would cause him to gain ten, maybe twenty pounds of belly fat and possibly become insulin-resistant. Instead, Voigt *lost* twenty-one pounds. His cholesterol and triglyceride levels dropped significantly, and even his resting blood glucose value—the linchpin in Atkins's theory of carbohydrate and weight gain—decreased. And like Mikkel Hindhede and Stanislaw Kon and Aniela Klein before him, Voigt suffered no loss of energy or functional capacity on an all-potato diet. Of course, as a paid potato advocate, he might not have admitted to having felt unwell on the diet even if he had. But Voigt seemed honest about the negatives, admitting, for example, that he was sick to death of eating potatoes long before the stunt ended.

Voigt was also forthright in confessing the one notable side effect of the diet. A habitual snorer, Voigt stopped snoring on the first night of his diet and did not snore again until the night after it ended. Who knew?

The Myth of Mechanisms as Outcomes

In bygone times, foods were judged by the health outcomes that resulted from them. People knew nothing about what happened inside the body to connect food inputs with health outputs. This has changed. The tools and technologies of science have allowed us to observe in microscopic detail how individual foods are processed and used by the body. Some of these processes have been identified as mechanisms through which positive or negative health outcomes result over time. Yet it has proven rather difficult in many cases to link individual foods to specific health outcomes through these mechanisms. The reason is that each food has numerous short-term effects on the body. A given food may therefore be healthful overall even if one of its short-term effects has been tied to negative health outcomes. But the human preference for black-and-white thinking about food has inspired many people to forget about health outcomes and to pass absolute judgment on foods based solely on their association with a "bad" mechanism.

More than a few healthy foods have been unfairly victimized by this tendency, none more than the potato. Before the rise of nutritional science, potato eaters in the real world knew that potatoes were good for them. Then the glycemic index was invented, and some folks decided that all high-glycemic foods, including the potato, were bad. It did not matter that an immediate spike in blood glucose after a meal was not inherently damaging to the body. It did not matter that eating (non-fried) potatoes was not associated with any negative long-term health consequences. What mattered was that, in theory, eating potatoes *ought* to be unhealthy.

This theory, which is based on the mistake of treating mechanisms as outcomes, has brought the potato's reputation so low that nutrition scientists working for the U.S. government have tried to prevent schoolchildren from eating potatoes and other vegetables, instead of fried foods, and were enthusiastically supported in this effort by many nutrition-conscious parents, perhaps including some who were very close to you.

It's a strange world we live in.

8

Eat Bad, Look Good

The cover story of the August 17, 2009 issue of *Time* magazine was provocatively titled "Why Exercise Won't Make You Thin." Written by *Time* staffer John Cloud, the article reported (with evident relish) that, despite what the public had been told a million times, exercise was not an effective way to lose weight. The reason, Cloud explained, was a newly recognized phenomenon called the *compensation effect*.

"The basic problem," he wrote, "is that while it's true that exercise burns calories and that you must burn calories to lose weight, exercise has another effect: it can stimulate hunger. That causes us to eat more, which in turn can negate the weight-loss benefits we just accrued. Exercise, in other words, isn't necessarily helping us lose weight. It may even be making it harder."

One of several respected scientists whom Cloud interviewed for his article put the matter even more bluntly, telling him, "In general, for weight loss, exercise is pretty useless." Just how useless was demonstrated in an experiment conducted by researchers at Louisiana State University. More than 300 sedentary, overweight women were separated into four groups. One group exercised under supervision for one hour and twelve minutes per week for six months. This was the "light exercise" group. Another eighty-five women were placed in the "moderate exercise" group, which worked out for two hours and sixteen minutes per week. The women who drew the short straw made up a "heavy exercise group," which exercised for three hours and fourteen minutes every week. The remaining ninety-four women comprised a control group that did not exercise. All of the subjects were asked to make no changes to their diet during the six-month intervention.

Women in all four groups (including the non-exercising control group, for some reason) lost a little weight, but the subjects in the heavy exercise group didn't lose any more weight than the women in the light exercise group and lost *less* weight than the subjects in the moderate exercise group. The authors of the study concluded that all of the additional exercise that the women in the heavy exercise group did served only to increase their appetite and make them eat more, counteracting the calorie-burning effect of the extra exercise.

Other research cited in Cloud's article suggested that working out might also thwart weight loss—and even promote weight *gain*—by making people less active than they would otherwise be during the rest of the day. Talk about a double-whammy of unintended consequences! If those forty minutes you spend on the treadmill at 24-Hour Fitness aren't already fully negated by the Starbucks Frappuccino you drink as a reward on the way home, then they will be when you decide you're too exhausted to walk the dog that evening.

"In short," Cloud summarized, "it's what you eat, not how hard you try to work it off, that matters more in losing weight."

This was shocking news to most *Time* readers in 2009. (It was also wonderful news, I'm sure, to the many who took it as license to remain sedentary.) But today the idea that exercise is not an effective way to lose weight is widely accepted. Anyone who has hired a personal trainer or read about weight loss on Yahoo! Health in the last several years knows that the formula for weight loss is "10 percent exercise, 90 percent diet."

Or is it? Not everyone who read Cloud's article bought what he was selling. The strongest skeptics were those who had themselves lost large amounts of weight with exercise and who therefore were living proof that exercise *can* make a person thin. Among the skeptics whose personal experience contradicted Cloud's thesis was the guy who wrote the words you are now reading. My case is doubly confounding for the claim that "exercise is pretty useless" because I lost sixty pounds by taking up aerobic exercise after previously *gaining* seventy pounds by *giving up* aerobic exercise.

It all started when I was seventeen years old. Throughout my entire life to that point I had never met a person who was skinnier than the scrawny youth I saw in the mirror every day. When I entered the twelfth grade I stood six feet, one inch (my current height) and weighed 138 pounds. My body mass index was 18.2, placing me in the category of the underweight. A genetic predisposition was probably mainly responsible for my emaciation, but I also ran forty miles a week for cross-country and track.

I hated my gaunt face and bony body. Worse than the teasing of my buddies was my inability to attract the caliber of girls I was attracted to. So when cross country season ended in November of my last year of high school, I launched upon a quest to bulk up. I stopped running cold turkey, took up weightlifting, and ate as much as I could. My plan succeeded beyond my wildest hopes. In ten weeks I gained thirty-four pounds. The only catch was that only half of the weight was muscle; the other half was blubber.

At first I wasn't alarmed. The flab was an amusing novelty— a trifling side effect of a problem solved. I recall entertaining my friends by hiding three golf balls between rolls of belly fat. I laughed right along with them, more delighted by my new muscles than I was embarrassed by my budding love handles. In any case, I was confident that the fat rolls would vanish just as quickly as they had appeared when I started running again to prepare for my freshman season on the Haverford College cross country team. But in the end I chose girls over running. And the very instant I made that decision, the novelty of my sloppy belly wore off. Having cast aside the only way I knew to get rid of it, I realized I was disgusted by it.

Several months of hoping the thing would go away on its own produced no results. Instead, I continued to gain weight. As before, the added mass was roughly half muscle (I continued to lift weights) and half blubber. I graduated weighing 206 pounds. By then I had grown heavy-metal hair down to my shoulder blades. I looked like a professional wrestler from the 1970s. I would have preferred to look like a fitness model of the present day, but I couldn't muster the discipline to say "no" to fried cheese cutlets at the cafeteria or drink less beer or eat less late-night pizza. I was powerless in the face of such temptations. Lacking the will to even *try* to lose weight by eating better, I just got bigger and bigger.

I might still be fat today if changing my diet had been my only option for losing weight. But fate gave me another option. When I was four years out of college, I decided to train for a triathlon. My goal was not to lose weight but to have fun and test myself. I had gotten a job as an editor at a triathlon magazine and found myself immersed in a culture that reawakened my passion for endurance sports. For the first time in almost a decade, I felt that old urge to race. So I stopped lifting weights and started swimming, bicycling, and running, often twice a day in preparation for the race. In just six weeks, I lost about twenty pounds despite a big spike in appetite that caused me to eat even more than I had been eating already. When I toed the starting line of my first marathon two years later, I was down to 150 pounds. Fifteen years further on, I still run marathons and I am still under 160.

I do eat much better now—and I specifically mean *better*, not *less*—which hasn't hurt. But I don't depend on healthy eating to stay lean. I rely on my training. When I'm working out two to three hours a day in preparation for a long triathlon or a marathon, I can eat pretty much nonstop without gaining an ounce. But when my workout habit is curtailed for any reason, I fatten up quickly even as I continue to eat carefully.

Given this background, you can imagine how incredulous I was when I read John Cloud's article in *Time* magazine. I felt the kind of exasperation Neil Armstrong might have felt if he had overheard a conversation between two people who agreed that the moon landing had been staged. I suppose if I were the *only* person who had ever lost a lot of weight through exercise, it wouldn't matter how absurd Cloud's argument looked to my eyes. But I am not alone—not by a long shot. In my personal and professional orbits, I routinely meet other people who have lost large amounts of weight the same way I did.

One of them is Fred Lechuga, whom I met through Facebook a few years back. Unlike me, Fred was born with a biological disposition toward obesity. His whole extended family was overweight, and by the time he was a year old he was obese himself. At the age of twenty-five, he weighed 360 pounds—and he was only five foot six.

When Fred became a father, he decided enough was enough and he set about losing weight. He changed his diet, but not drastically. Like me, Fred lacked the motivation to eat less, so he just tried to eat a little better. For example, instead of having two

McDonald's Egg McMuffins for breakfast on the way to work, he ate a four-egg omelet with veggies and cheese at home.

Nobody had ever told Fred that "exercise is pretty useless" for weight loss, so he went ahead and relied mainly on exercise to lose weight. He started with hybrid workouts that consisted of thirty or forty minutes of weightlifting followed by twenty or thirty minutes of jogging on a treadmill. After a while, Fred realized that the weightlifting wasn't really doing much good, whereas he kind of enjoyed the running, so he quit the first and doubled down on the other. Before long, he was running ninety minutes to two hours a day. Within a year he had lost more than 100 pounds.

There are a couple of clues that Fred's running, more than his dietary changes, deserve credit for his transformation. First, a full decade after his initial weight loss, and long after he had settled into his new diet, Fred decided to run a marathon. During the four months he trained for it, he lost another twenty-three pounds, bringing his total weight loss to 170 pounds. Second, when Fred gets injured and can't run, he puts on fat so quickly, it's like a time-lapse video.

I could cite many other cases like Fred's, but I trust I've made my point. The world is full of people who are living proof that exercise has the power to stimulate major weight loss. As we've seen, however, the scientific evidence appears to prove the opposite. This disparity is explained in part by individuality. Although the average amount of weight loss is usually modest in experiments like the one John Cloud highlighted in his *Time* article, some of the subjects lose a lot of weight while others lose little or none and still others actually gain weight. It seems there is a large degree of individual variation in the effect of exercise on appetite. Some people eat as few as two or three extra calories for every ten calories they sweat off. Others compensate for every single calorie burned in workouts. Scientists have also identified genes that render some people highly responsive to the fat-burning potential of exercise, and other genes that make their unlucky possessors (known as "nonresponders") resistant to it. So perhaps the title of John Cloud's *Time* article should have been "Why Exercise Won't Make *Some People* Thin."

But there's another factor to consider. In the LSU study that Cloud described, the members of the so-called *heavy* exercise group worked out just twenty-seven minutes a day at an intensity of just 50 percent of their maximum breathing capacity (or "VO_2max"), which corresponds to a slow walk for the typical overweight beginning exerciser. Compare that to the ninety minutes or more of fairly intense exercise that Fred Lechuga does almost every day.

It's simple math. The "heavy exercisers" in the LSU study burned about 130 calories per day through exercise, or a little more than a twelve-ounce soda's worth. Fred Lechuga burns closer to *1,500* calories a day with his running, or roughly the number of calories in a four-egg omelet with cheese and veggies, a turkey sandwich, and two cups of boiled spaghetti with tomato sauce.

I'm not suggesting that the scientists who study the effects of exercise on body weight intentionally set up exercise for failure by requiring pitifully small amounts of pathetically easy exercise. They are simply bowing to a practical necessity. An obese couch potato who is thrown headlong into an exercise program that requires her to work out for ninety minutes to two hours a day at 70 percent of VO_2max is bound to get injured. These people must be gently eased into exercise. But doing so creates a false appearance that exercise is ineffective for weight loss. To see that exercise truly can stimulate weight loss, you have to look at the folks like Fred and me who have fallen in love with endurance sports and don't mind devoting a lot of time to working out, day after day, month after month, year after year.

The fact of the matter is that anyone—even a nonresponder—can lose weight through exercise. It just takes a lot of exercise. But here's another thing: it is almost impossible to *maintain* weight loss without exercise. In Chapter 5 we saw that a big commitment to exercise is the single best predictor of successful weight-loss maintenance. When people lose weight through diet alone, they almost invariably regain all of the lost pounds and often end up heavier than before. The point of losing weight is to lose it *permanently*. While dieting is, for most people, more effective than exercise in triggering weight loss, exercise is more effective than diet in maintaining a stable body weight following weight loss, which makes dieting without exercise rather pointless.

The effectiveness of exercise as an instrument for weight maintenance is most strikingly apparent in competitive endurance athletes. There is a popular assumption that, as a group, obese individuals consume the most food. In fact, competitive endurance athletes typically consume substantially more calories than even the morbidly obese, which is interesting, because endurance athletes are also the leanest segment of society. That's right: the *leanest* people on earth eat the most food. How is this possible? Lots of exercise.

During the 2008 Beijing Summer Olympics, it was revealed that swimmer Michael Phelps ate 12,000 calories a day during peak training periods, or more than four times the number of calories the average American male eats. (And remember, the average American male is overweight.) What's more, almost all of these calories came from foods that a nutritionist would classify as garbage. Phelps's typical day's menu consisted of a five-egg omelet, two cups of coffee, three fried egg sandwiches, three chocolate chip pancakes, french toast with powdered sugar, a bowl of grits, two pounds of pasta, two ham and cheese sandwiches with extra mayonnaise, an entire pizza, and 2,000 calories in energy drinks. Phelps later claimed that the 12,000-calorie figure was inflated, but he never disputed the menu itself.

Despite these junky eating habits, Phelps was so lean that the outlines of his abdominal muscles showed through the skin of his tummy. The reason he looked so good despite eating so badly was that he swam four hours a day and lifted weights every other day, incinerating every calorie he ate except those that were used to preserve his lean form.

Later in his career, with cleaner-eating rivals threatening his supremacy, Phelps tidied up his diet a bit, replacing fried-egg sandwiches with oatmeal and fresh fruit at breakfast and swapping pizza for lean meats and vegetables at the dinner table. Nowadays most elite endurance athletes eat far more healthily than even the reformed Michael Phelps did. But in past generations, diets that looked more like the original Michael Phelps diet were the norm among swimmers, cyclists, and especially runners. The heroes of the so-called "running boom" in the 1970s took pride in being able to eat whatever the hell they wanted without paying a price. Bill Rodgers, winner of four Boston marathons and four New York City marathons, famously filled up on mayonnaise, sugary breakfast cereals, chocolate-chip cookies, snack chips, soft drinks, and gin-and-tonics.

The dietary slogan of the running boomers was drawn from the cult novel *Once a Runner*, self-published in 1978. Author John L. Parker, Jr. wrote, "If the furnace is hot enough, anything burns, even Big Macs." That phrase—"If the furnace is hot enough, anything burns"—has remained a catchphrase of junk-eating competitive runners ever since.

Some runners have even taken to heart the part about Big Macs. In 2011 a runner from Palatine, Illinois, named Joe D'Amico ate only McDonald's food during the last thirty days of his training for the Los Angeles Marathon. Not only did he finish the race, but he finished twenty-eighth overall in a field of 20,000 runners with a time of 2:36:14. A few years earlier, film-maker Morgan Spurlock had eaten only McDonald's for thirty days *without* exercising and had gained twenty-five pounds. Yet when D'Amico combined the same diet with intensive exercise he was fit enough to run more than ten miles per hour for 26.2 miles.

It takes more than a lean body composition to run a 2:36 marathon as Joe D'Amico did, much less a pair of 2:09 marathons as Bill Rodgers did, or to swim a 400 IM in 4:03 as Michael Phelps did. It also requires extremely high levels of all-around fitness and health. So it would appear that much more than a low body weight is attainable despite a mediocre diet given sufficient exercise, at least in those who are fairly young. Science confirms that exercise indeed possesses remarkable powers to neutralize the negative health effects of imperfect eating.

For starters, exercise cancels out the costs of eating too much fat. After a person eats a high-fat meal there is a sudden influx of fat molecules into the blood stream. Scientists call this phenomenon *postprandial lipemia* and they believe it contributes to the development of atherosclerosis. The amount of fat that appears in the blood after a high-fat meal is significantly reduced when exercise is undertaken either before or after the meal. This benefit of exercise is especially pronounced in physically fit individuals who exercise regularly.

Exercise also neutralizes the bad effects of eating too much carbohydrate. The sudden influx of carbohydrate into the blood stream that occurs after a high-carbohydrate meal causes the pancreas to release insulin, which delivers much of that carbohydrate to adipose tissue, where it is converted to fat. Exercise protects against this consequence of eating carbohydrate-rich meals by increasing insulin sensitivity in muscle tissue, which becomes a kind of sponge that soaks up carbs, leaving less to be stored as fat. A single workout increases insulin sensitivity for twenty-four hours. So if you work out every day, you can eat more or less all the carbs you like without worrying about getting fat.

Exercise even makes up for not eating enough vitamins. Research involving laboratory animals has shown that regular exercise completely counteracts certain health consequences (such as susceptibility to free radical damage) that are associated with a diet deficient in vitamins and minerals. There is limited evidence that exercise makes up for nutrient deficiencies in humans too. In 2005 researchers from the University of Copenhagen analyzed the diet of twelve adolescent runners in Kenya. It was found to be deficient in six essential vitamins plus the minerals calcium and selenium. Despite the inadequacies, these young runners were healthy enough to perform at a world-class level.

A small number of human studies have attempted to directly address the following question: Who is healthier, a person who eats healthily and does not exercise, or a person who exercises and does not eat healthily? In 2007 researchers at the Washington University School of Medicine measured several cardiometabolic and cancer risk factors in three groups: sedentary vegans, runners on Western diets, and sedentary people on Western diets. (While veganism is not synonymous with healthy eating, the typical vegan diet is a lot healthier than the typical "Western" diet.) Almost all of the risk factors were found to be lower in both vegans and runners than in the control group.

If this study proves that a heavy exerciser with a mediocre diet is likely to be just as healthy as a nonexerciser with a very good diet, then it also proves the reverse. But the story doesn't end here, because exercise enhances health in other ways that diet does not.

Many people believe that a good diet with plenty of calcium ensures healthy bones. Not so. By far the most important contributor to bone health is weight-bearing exercise. You can eat all the calcium you want and your bones will be as brittle as Tinker Toys if all you do is lie in bed all day.

Exercise also does more than diet for brain health. A good diet can slow the rate at which the brain ages and loses functional capacity. But exercise actually reverses these processes, adding gray matter, boosting neuroplasticity, and heightening cognitive function.

Cardiorespiratory fitness itself—which is strongly affected by exercise but only weakly affected by diet—is not only a useful attribute for endurance athletes but is also an important health factor. Research has shown that cardiorespiratory fitness is a strong predictor of longevity across the lifespan, and in old age especially. Exercise is associated with a high level of cardiorespiratory fitness in the elderly, but healthy eating is not.

Then there's the matter of how you *feel* when you're really fit. Health is typically defined in the negative, as the absence of disease, but I prefer to define health positively, in terms of the functional capacity of the body's many systems and of the organism as a whole. A good diet does not increase functional capacity; it merely enables the body to fully exploit existing capacity. Exercise has the power to drastically enhance the functional capacity of nearly every system of the body. At rest, a physically fit individual is aware of the latent capacity within him, sensing it as a kind of overflowing vitality.

It is often said that life is a marathon, and not without reason. Everyday life on earth today is a test of endurance. When you have the energy to run 26.2 miles, daily life is a cakewalk. You feel like a comic book hero as you sail through the quotidian routine of commuting, working, fixing meals, helping your kids with their homework, and all the rest. You can't get that feeling from eating like a saint and never leaving your recliner.

The Best of Both Worlds

In consideration of all this, you might now wonder if the heaviest exercisers, including competitive endurance athletes, should even bother trying to eat well. We've already seen that many elite endurance athletes of past generations decided healthy eating was not worth the trouble. But the level of competition is higher today, and athletes need to exploit every little advantage. Most professional endurance athletes in our time eat very healthily—in an agonistic way—because it makes a small difference in a sport that is now all about small differences.

Body fat percentage is one of the strongest predictors of racing performance among elite endurance athletes. The winner of any given race is likely to have a tiny bit less fat on his or her body than the second-place finisher. Elite endurance athletes cannot rely on favorable genes and hard training alone to get as lean and fast as they can possibly be. A good diet is required to rid them of those last few ounces—or grams—of dead weight.

There have been some noteworthy examples of professional endurance athletes who appeared to be getting away with bad eating until they started eating better. Consider Chris Horner. Throughout a long career as a professional cyclist, Horner fueled himself with Cokes, Snickers bars, breakfast burritos, donuts, Little Debbie brownies, Swiss Rolls, hold-the-veggies sandwiches, potato chips, and fast food. Despite his terrible diet, Horner excelled as a climbing specialist and he won a lot of races. He saw no reason to fix what did not appear to be broken.

Then a crash in the 2009 Tour of California left Horner unable to ride for two weeks. Knowing he could ill afford to gain several pounds during a fortnight without exercise, he decided to finally give better eating a try. Horner cut way down on the burgers and sweets and introduced a few fruits and vegetables to his diet. Even with these changes his diet remained far from perfect, but they had an impact. Instead of gaining weight while laid up, Horner began to lose weight. When he got back in the saddle he continued to lean out, eventually losing ten pounds of fat he hadn't even known were there. Soon he was climbing better than ever. In 2010, when Horner was thirty-eight years old, an age at which most cyclists are either already retired or contemplating retirement, he won his first major European stage race. Three years later and still eating carefully, Horner became the oldest champion of a Grand Tour, winning the Vuelta a España just weeks before he turned forty-two.

Even if it's just a few pounds of performance-sapping excess body fat, there is always some cost to eating poorly. Other potential costs include iron deficiency anemia, stress fractures, and frequent upper respiratory tract infections—common health problems among competitive endurance athletes that are especially common among those with poor diets.

The most dreaded runner's health crisis is overtraining syndrome, a form of chronic fatigue that takes months to shake off and may also be affected by diet. Is it a coincidence that the runner who once bragged of having the "world's worst diet" was felled by chronic fatigue in the middle of his career? Anthony Famiglietti was raised on a diet that included no fruits or vegetables except for pizza sauce. He continued to eat garbage throughout his college years and well into a career as a professional runner. "Fam" survived entirely on fast-food burgers and fries, breakfast cereals, macaroni and cheese, pizza, and candy. And he was proud of it. In his self-produced DVD *Run Like Hell*, Fam boasted that he did not know what broccoli tasted like.

"My whole thing is if the furnace is burning hot enough, you can throw anything in there," Fam said with a nod to John L. Parker, Jr., in an NPR interview. "You can just eat whatever you want."

There seemed to be no reason to change. Famiglietti achieved outstanding results despite his bad eating. He won three national championships, a World University Games gold medal, and a Pan-Am Games bronze medal in his specialty, the 3000-meter steeplechase. In 2006, at age twenty-seven, he had a career year, winning the USA 5-km road title and setting personal best times in three track events.

The very next year, Fam's body fell apart. First he struggled to a fourth-place finish in the 2007 USA national championships steeplechase final. Then he shut down completely. A crippling fatigue laid him flat. No matter how much sleep he got, he still needed more. No matter how much he cut back on his training, he felt no better. For two weeks Fam could not even run a full mile without pausing for a walk break. A friend and dietitian convinced Fam it was time to find out what broccoli tasted like.

The ailing runner completely transformed his diet, along with other elements of his lifestyle (taking up meditation and spiritual reading, for example). In 2008, Fam was back and better than ever. He won the Olympic Trials steeplechase and set a new personal-best time in Beijing. By then he had learned that his chronic fatigue had been caused by the Epstein-Barr virus, but he felt so much better on his new diet that he was not at all tempted to seize upon the revised diagnosis as an excuse to backslide. Like those recovered alcoholics who become alcohol counselors, Famiglietti now preaches the gospel of healthy eating, sometimes visiting natural food markets to discuss his newfound love of quinoa, sugar-free peanut butter, and "dark fruits" (plums, red grapes, cherries, açai berries, etc.).

The You-Are-What-You-Eat Myth

Exercise is the great equalizer of diets. Any diet, good or bad, will affect the body of a person who exercises very differently than it affects the body of a person who does not exercise. Regular physical activity ensures that the nutrients a person consumes are put to the best possible use. Exercisers may indeed get more out of an average diet than non-exercisers get out of a good one.

Yet exercise only intensifies a tendency that is manifest in the body even at rest—a tendency to fabricate the same final product out of whatever raw materials it is given. The body is able to "zero out" small to moderate differences in food choices and eating patterns—in other words, to derive the same level of health from diverse ways of eating. Inside each of us there are scores of built-in mechanisms that work to maintain a preferred physiological homeostasis despite varying nutritional resources. If you eat more salt, the excess will be excreted in urine. If you reduce your carbohydrate intake, your body will create more carbs (and carb substitutes) from the fats in your diet. Evolution has designed the human body to achieve its required output from a variety of different inputs, and this is one reason there is no "best" diet for everyone.

The most hackneyed, if not the oldest, dietary cliché is the saying, "You are what you eat." So familiar is this axiom that we seldom consider its true meaning. What it suggests is that our health is rigidly determined by the specific foods and nutrients we put in our bodies. It says that if two people put the same foods in their body, they will have the same level of health. And if two people put different foods in their body, they are likely to experience different health outcomes. We are *entirely*, *only*, and *exactly* what we eat.

The healthy-diet cults unanimously subscribe to this principle. You could read a hundred diet-cult books, attend a hundred diet-cult lectures, and watch a hundred diet-cult videos without ever seeing or hearing anything that contradicted the essential meaning of "You are what you eat." This is only to be expected. After all, the diet cults are in business to convince us that we can attain maximum health only if we eat what they tell us to eat.

But in fact we are not what we eat. We are *what our bodies do with* what we eat. If the body's basic metabolism zeroes out small to moderate differences in diet, exercise neutralizes moderate to large differences. It is like a great sculptor who can fashion the same beautiful form out of various materials, including some of indifferent quality. Exercise is not a license to eat any which way, but we can't attain maximum health without it, and with it we can attain maximum health through an infinite variety of healthy diets—no cult required.

9

Coffee, Chocolate, and Wine

A sign located just inside the front entrance of the East West Café in Sebastopol, California, enjoins visitors to "Buy local! Support Sebastopol Business." A smaller sign located near the first one invites arriving diners to seat themselves. On a bright Saturday morning in the summer of 2012, my wife, Nataki, and I chose a small table against a wall.

Nataki ordered Eggs Benedict and orange juice. I ordered a Veggie Benedict, an all-fruit smoothie, and a mug of "Taylor Maid Organic Sustainable" coffee. Patrons of the East West Café can buy nothing more local than the last of these items. At the time of our visit, the Taylor Maid Farms roasting facility was located two blocks from where we sat. (It has since moved a couple of miles away.)

When the coffee was poured, I eyed it with concern. Its color was the wan mahogany of mediocre java. I closed my mouth and breathed in—and my concern deepened. The vaguely burnt scent that filled my nostrils was all too familiar from a million previously visited breakfast joints serving cheap roasts to eaters who dumped so much Sweet-n-Low in their mugs that it hardly mattered what they were drinking.

A sip confirmed my fears. The coffee certainly wasn't bad. If I had just stumbled upon this place randomly I would have been pleasantly surprised. But it wasn't what I had come all this way for.

I do not call myself a coffee connoisseur. A connoisseur can say more about a sip of Italian roast than I can say about an entire meal. Nor am I a coffee snob. I drink Starbucks and no-name coffees frequently with nary a complaint. But I do love coffee. I started drinking it when I was twenty-five years old and living in the Haight-Ashbury neighborhood of San Francisco. My girlfriend of five and a half years had recently dumped me and I was despondent. I was riding the bus to my awful temp job stacking boxes at the headquarters of Jamba Juice one morning when I spied a small newspaper item about a new study reporting that coffee drinkers were less likely to commit suicide than was the average person. The next morning, before I caught the bus, I bought a cup of coffee at an independent café on the southwest corner of Haight and Ashbury. A couple of the baristas there were recovering heroin addicts. The stuff they served was as thick and dark as motor oil and as potent as rocket fuel. To this day I have not had a stronger cup of joe than my first—and I drank it black, because I wasn't drinking it for the taste. But I liked it. And ever since then I have preferred saucy brews that slap me across the face.

Whenever I travel I try to find out where the best local coffee is served and sample it. On this particular weekend Nataki and I had driven three hours from our home in California's Central Valley to Sonoma County to eat and drink our way through wine country—something we manage to do once every few years. My research into local coffee roasters had brought us to the East West Café.

We paid for our breakfast and left. Knowing that even the best grinds can be ruined by indifferent brewing, I begged Nataki's indulgence and led her down the street to the Taylor Maid Farms headquarters. Primarily a roasting facility, with big loading bays and cargo vans parked out front, the Taylor Maid building had a tiny café of its own tucked into a corner. The company was founded in 1993 by Chris Martin, owner of the eponymous farm, and Mark Inman, a master roaster who studied winemaking before he got turned on to coffee. In 2005, Inman explained his leap from wine to coffee to a *New York Times* reporter.

"I was invited to a coffee tasting," he said. "I thought I would fly into the room and dazzle everyone with my palate. Instead, I left there completely humbled. So far as taste is concerned, coffee offered everything that wine offered and more."

As Nataki and I entered the cramped café, which served not a crumb of food, I noticed a sticker pasted to the glass front door identifying the establishment as a "Go Local—Sonoma County Member." Inside we found a couple of hipster baristas who greeted us with diffident nods but who came alive when I started to pepper them with questions about their coffees. The more senior of the two, who confessed without embarrassment to having come over recently from Starbucks, waxed poetic about his current employer's single-origin coffees, which are the coffee equivalent of the varietals and appellations that make wine connoisseurship not just possible but necessary. This was another topic Mark Inman had discussed in his *Times* interview.

"We are ready for consumers who come into the store and order single-origin coffees from a particular region of Panama," he said.

If such consumers existed seven years later, I was not one of them. At the risk of disappointing our barista, I ordered a cup of Red Rooster French Roast, a premium blend of several beans. It took five minutes to prepare using the pour-over method. The beans for my individual serving were scooped, weighed, and ground. The water was heated to a precise ninety-seven degrees. The hot water was then poured over a ceramic Hario dripper with a practiced circular motion. A cloth filter was used. The brew filtered through the grounds and into a glass flask that sat upon a kitchen scale, whose purpose was to ensure that my cup contained the ideal balance of coffee grounds and water.

When the performance was completed, I grabbed my mug and Nataki claimed her Farmhouse Decaf, and we walked outside to sit on cast-iron chairs and soak in the pure sunlight of a fast-warming July morning. My coffee was colored the blackest shade of brown and was rimmed with a butterscotch froth. The aroma seemed the platonic ideal of "coffee smell." I tasted it.

Again, I'm no connoisseur. But I can tell the difference between a good cup of coffee and a great one, between great and memorable. I've had a few memorable cups of coffee. And this was one of them.

Steaming Elixir

Unless you already know otherwise, you might assume that the first coffee drinkers were inhabitants of the island of Java. In fact, coffee is believed to have originated in Yemen, where people chewed coffee berries to get high before a Sufi Muslim named Muhammad al-Dhabhani came up with the idea of making a hot drink out of them in the middle of the fifteenth century. Al-Dhabhani and other Sufis used the beverage initially to keep themselves awake through all-night religious ceremonies.

In the early 1500s, coffee consumption spread throughout the Muslim world, where it was embraced as an acceptable alternative to forbidden alcoholic drinks. European visitors to Cairo and Mecca and other cities where coffeehouses had become as common as pubs were in European cities took note of the phenomenon and brought the custom back home. By the middle of the seventeenth century, coffee fever was spreading like the plague in London, Amsterdam, and elsewhere.

Early adopters of coffee drinking were not won over by the drink's taste. Beans were usually lightly pan-roasted—a method that does not bring out a lot of flavor. Arab coffee drinkers triple-boiled their mixtures of water and grinds to produce greater richness, but English coffeehouses of the time stored cold coffee in big kegs and reheated it for serving, and thus its flavor was described by some as a mixture of soot and old shoes. Only when modern roasting and brewing methods were perfected did coffee become as tasty as the best cups are today. And not until the rise of the so-called "Third Wave" in the 1990s did a bona fide connoisseur culture coalesce around coffee.

The reason coffee caught on before it even tasted good is that it contains a drug, caffeine, that produces a high. Caffeine's chemical structure is similar to that of adenosine, a compound that is produced naturally by the body and functions as a neuromodulator. When caffeine molecules attach themselves to adenosine receptors in the brain, a coffee drinker experiences sensations of alertness and euphoria. These sensations do more than jolt us into readiness for a new day in the morning, or any other time we need a pick-me-up. In 2011, researchers at the Harvard School of Public Health reported that habitual coffee drinkers were up to 20 percent less likely to suffer from depression than were those who did not drink coffee. Fifteen years earlier, another Harvard study—the very one I read about so serendipitously on a bus in San Francisco—found that heavy coffee drinkers were up to 40 percent less likely to kill themselves.

When I learned of and personally benefited from coffee's mental health effects in 1996, coffee and caffeine were widely considered to be unhealthy. That was nothing new. The healthfulness of coffee has been debated for as long as it has existed, and only within the past twenty years has science settled the matter in coffee's favor. Seventeenth-century coffee haters claimed that the drink caused impotence, anorexia, blood disorders, and moral depravity. But twenty-first-century science has shown that coffee drinkers are healthier than coffee non-drinkers in a variety of ways and that the heaviest coffee drinkers benefit the most. Coffee fiends are less likely than others to develop heart disease, diabetes, dementia, some cancers, liver disease, Parkinson's disease, and (again) depression. Coffee drinkers may even live longer than abstainers. A 2012 study published in the *New England Journal of Medicine* found that, within a population of more than 400,000 men and women, regular coffee drinkers were 10 percent less likely to die during a thirteen-year period. Scientists have also learned that it's not just the caffeine content of coffee that enhances health, but also its antioxidants.

Athletes love coffee because it enhances athletic performance—so much so that caffeine use is regulated by the International Olympic Committee. Caffeine improves speed and strength by accelerating the transmission of electrical signals from the brain to the muscles. It improves endurance by reducing perception of effort—that is, by making sustained efforts such as marathon running feel easier.

Despite the completely one-sided avalanche of evidence of coffee's healthfulness, there remain some dietary ascetics who insist that coffee is pernicious. A number of healthy-diet cults, including the Atkins diet, the Zone Diet, the candida diet, and various detox diets, forbid or strictly limit coffee consumption. Each offers its own particular physiological rationale for doing so, but one suspects that underneath these disparate reasons lies an age-old puritanical presumption that a thing people consume for pleasure can't possibly be good for them.

Pursuit of Pleasure

Nataki and I finished our coffee and drove back to the Hilton Sonoma Wine Country, a campus-style hotel whose several separate buildings were all named after wines. Our room was in the Chablis building. An apartment complex just up the hill from the Hilton was called The Vineyards. The largest industry in Sonoma County is winemaking. The second biggest is wine tourism. You feel like you're in a giant wine theme park when you visit.

After freshening up in the air-conditioned comfort of our junior suite, we departed again. At eleven o'clock in the morning, it was already almost—but not quite—too hot to drop the top of Nataki's convertible. A ten-minute drive brought us to a small retail plaza that contained a little shop called Recherché du Plaisir (French for "Pursuit of Pleasure"). A modest sign above the entrance advertised "Chocolates, Confections & Sweet Bites." We stepped inside.

Recherché du Plaisir had opened just seven months earlier, and everything still looked new. A model Eiffel Tower stood against the front wall. A small framed black-and-white photographic print hung from another wall. It depicted a couple of stylish Parisian flappers sipping coffee at a little outdoor table. These details went unnoticed until later. Our eyes were drawn first to the mouthwatering displays of truffles and macaroons at either end of a long serving counter. Behind the counter stood Lucy Gustafson, a smiling, matronly woman in her mid-forties and the proprietress of the establishment.

I had emailed ahead to tell Lucy that my wife and I were interested in a chocolate-tasting experience similar to the wine tastings that are the stock-in-trade of wine tourism in Sonoma. I was also interested in hearing her ideas about chocolate. An anonymous quotation on her shop's website gave me a pretty good sense of Lucy's perspective: "Life should not be a journey to the grave with the intention of arriving safely in an attractive, well-preserved body, but rather to skid in sideways, chocolate in one hand, wine in the other, body thoroughly used up, totally worn out and screaming, 'Woo-hoo! What a ride.'"

During the half hour Nataki and I spent inside the shop, I learned that Lucy was raised in Forestville, a small town just west of Santa Rosa. Her father was a schoolteacher. When Lucy was nine years old, the family rented out their home and relocated to France for six months. She fell in love with the country and was particularly impressed by the French mastery of the art of living.

"I think the Europeans have it right," she told us. "It's fine to work hard but you also need to play hard and enjoy your life."

When Lucy came home from France she immediately began to plot her return to the Old World. As soon as she was old enough to work, she took jobs cleaning the homes of neighbors, saving as much of her small income as she could. One of these neighbors happened to be making chocolate truffles one day as Lucy scrubbed and vacuumed. She was mesmerized by the process, which to her eyes had all the grace and refinement of a ballroom dance. When the job was completed, Lucy was rewarded with a sample.

"I couldn't believe how much flavor could exist in such a small package," she said, looking as though she could almost taste it still.

At seventeen, Lucy got her chance to go back to Europe, touring Germany on a bicycle with a friend. Four years later she crossed the Atlantic once more for a backpacking trip. Lucy then settled into a career in the travel industry, having chosen it mainly for the travel perks. In her free time she made chocolates to give away as gifts. Her truffles were a huge hit at her twenty-fifth high school reunion. Some of her old schoolmates urged her to go into business. Impulsively, Lucy decided to go for it. She enrolled in Ecole Chocolat's Professional Chocolatier Program, where she perfected her craft, and upon graduating she invested her life savings in creating Recherché du Plaisir. Less than a year after opening the door, she was already ahead of her schedule to break even.

I asked Lucy to tell us about her chocolates.

"I don't do bean to bar," she said, assuming I knew what that meant. "I buy my chocolate in bulk from Ghirardelli because they're a good California company and also from Gytard because they're all about fair trade. And I use Callebaut as my finishing chocolate."

Just then a young woman charged breathlessly into the store.

"I saw the sign," she announced, referring to a portable sign that Lucy's husband, Mike, was waving around out close to the freeway. "I said, 'Oh, boy! Finally something that's not See's!'" The woman then turned to Nataki and me, as though sniffing tourists, and quickly added, "I support local."

She quickly picked out a selection of truffles and hurried away. Lucy turned her attention back to us, and I asked her what I should focus on when tasting a fine chocolate.

"First of all, it should start to melt in your hand within a few seconds," she said. "The cheaper waxy ones don't."

I'd never thought of that.

"It should also have a nice sheen," she continued. "Texture is just as important as taste. When you bite in, you should get a nice snap and the truffle shouldn't be grainy. As for the flavor: the simpler, the better."

My wife and I studied the various offerings in the truffle case and decided to start with the AC/DC, which was described as "Ancho chile swimming in dark chocolate with spices and a whisper of fire."

I received a sample on my palm, noted its healthy sheen, and gave it a few seconds to start melting on my palm. I took a bite, and my knees nearly buckled.

"It's exquisite," I said. "It's hard to believe these are good for you."

"Mine aren't," Lucy said proudly. "To get the health benefits you need to eat something that's at least 72 percent cacao. I only go up to 68 percent because anything above that is too crumbly." She paused. "My chocolates are strictly for pleasure."

Food of the Gods

Chocolate was, in a sense, the original coffee—and it too contains caffeine. As long ago as 1500 B.C.E. native Central Americans figured out how to brew a deliciously bitter and intoxicating drink with inedible cacao beans. The first chocolate drinkers interpreted its unique flavor and mood-lifting effect as magical properties of divine origin. Like the first coffee drinkers, they used the concoction in religious ceremonies.

The Spanish explorer Hernán Cortés became the first European to drink chocolate when he landed in Mexico in 1518. He wasn't too impressed. Chocolate became popular in the Old World only after someone came up with the idea of sweetening it with honey or sugar. Solid chocolate did not come along until 1828, when a Dutch chemist developed a way to make a powder from chocolate liquor. Solid milk chocolate was introduced by Henri Nestlé in 1866, and the first chocolate candies were brought to market by John Cadbury a couple of years later.

Liquid chocolate was considered to be nourishing, even medicinal, in seventeenth-century Europe. Only later, when most cacao was consumed in sugary candy bars, did chocolate lose its healthful reputation. Chocolate continued to be known as a deliciously bad-for-you indulgence until the 1990s. I am old enough to remember when health-conscious eaters ate carob as a "healthier" substitute for chocolate. But recent science has revealed that chocolate (or cacao, anyway) is indeed healthy, perhaps even medicinal.

The first studies of chocolate's health effects found that it had a favorable effect on blood platelet formation, a risk factor for heart disease. This effect was attributed to the high concentration of polyphenols, a class of antioxidant, in cacao. Subsequent studies demonstrated that regular chocolate consumption significantly reduced the risk of heart disease. Dark chocolate in particular has since been shown to lower blood pressure in the hypertensive, improve circulation, increase HDL ("good") cholesterol, reduce the risk of heart attack and stroke, and increase insulin sensitivity (thus reducing the risk for diabetes).

Recent research has even suggested that chocolate may prevent weight gain in some people. A 2012 study by researchers at the University of California, San Diego, found that middle-aged men and women who ate small amounts of chocolate five or more times per week weighed five to seven pounds less, on average, than did those who ate no chocolate.

The beneficial effects on mood and mental state, which the first chocolate drinkers most appreciated, have also been confirmed by science. Chocolate lovers often describe its immediate effect as drug-like, and it turns out there's a good reason for that. Chocolate stimulates opioid production in the brain, just like cocaine. But while chocolate is able to turn a bad mood into a good one, it is not able to make a good mood better. No wonder people who suffer from depression eat twice as much chocolate as others do.

Another difference between chocolate and coffee is that it's not the tiny amount of caffeine or any other chemicals in chocolate but the taste that generates happy feelings. Tasteless chocolate doesn't do the trick. This explains why the mood-lifting effect of a really tasty chocolate is instantaneous—and fleeting.

Thanks to media hyping and corporate opportunism, dark chocolate has been broadly embraced as a health food. But it remains forbidden or restricted in a number of healthy-diet cults, including the Paleo Diet and vegan diets.

A Smooth Finish

Nataki and I left Recherché du Plaisir with fifty-three dollars in truffles and with detailed instructions on how to care for them.

On our way out the door, I asked Lucy for a restaurant recommendation. We wanted to take our lunch somewhere on the lovely town square in Healdsburg. Lucy said something that sounded like "shark's teeth." I asked her to spell it out. "C-H-A-R-C-U-T-E-R-I-E." Before the day was out, I would learn that the word was French for "the art of making sausage and cured meats."

Thirty minutes later, Nataki and I were seated at a cozy window table inside the establishment Lucy had so confidently selected for us. We started off with the Charcuterie Plate: Rosette de Lyon salami, duck rillette, pork pepper paté, garlic salami, brie, olives, and cornichons. Nataki chose a Cobb salad as her entrée and I picked the Sonoma salad. Our plan was to eat lightly because we had an afternoon of wine tasting ahead of us.

Actually, we'd already started the wine tasting. Nataki sipped a Peterson Muscat Blanc "Home Farm" 2007 with her meal, while I made quick work of a Bluenose Chardonnay. Not only our wines but also many of the ingredients in our meals, our waitress proudly informed us, were locally sourced.

Having visited most of the local wineries on past trips, Nataki and I decided to do our wine tasting in the tasting rooms that were sprinkled around the square in Healdsburg. More drinking, less driving. Our first stop was Murphy-Goode. A vest-wearing young fellow with a charming lisp and a name badge that said "Max" served us the five wines on the tasting menu plus a few extras that he poured in a because-I-like-you sort of way. At our hotel the previous night, Nataki and I had boned up on how to taste wine like grownups. Finding a copy of *The California Directory of Fine Wineries* in the room, I read aloud the page titled "The Etiquette of Wine Tasting."

"After you are served," I declaimed, affecting a posh accent, "hold the stem of the glass with your thumb and as many fingers as you need to maintain control. Lift the glass up to the light and note the color and intensity of the wine. . . . Next, gently swirl the wine in the glass. Observe how much of the wine adheres to the sides of the glass. . . . Now, tip the glass to about a 45-degree angle, take a short sniff, and concentrate on the aromas. . . . Finally, take a sip and swirl the wine around your tongue, letting your taste buds pick up all the flavors. The wine may remind you of honey or cherries or mint—as with the 'nosing,' try to make as many associations as you can. Then spit the wine into the bucket on the counter."

I did all of these things at the Murphy-Goode tasting room except spit. I wasn't ready to be *that* grown-up. Nor was I trying to pass myself off as a veteran oenophile. I told Max right away that I knew nothing about wine. He responded by coaching us through each pouring, telling us exactly what we should expect to taste. But halfway through our flight, I asked him to stop. I wanted to see how well I could do on my own. The answer was: not well. My tasting experience quickly degenerated into a ridiculous charades-like guessing game.

"Vanilla?" I said after trying the 2006 Snake Eyes Zinfandel.

"Black raspberry," Max said. "Blackberry jam."

My subsequent guesses were even farther off the mark. Nataki and Max were having a pretty good laugh at my expense when we received our last sample, the 2008 Semillon Late Harvest. My eyes widened.

"Licorice!" I blurted. Max threw me a high-five.

"Yes!" he lisped. I bought a bottle.

Our next stop was La Crema, where the light buzz we had already acquired persuaded us to pay fifteen dollars apiece for the "Exclusive Flight" instead of five dollars for the "Introductory Flight." I gave up the guessing game and tried to taste everything mentioned in the notes we were given. Even with the aid of suggestion, I could never identify more than one of the six or seven flavors I was told to expect. The 2008 Carneros Hills Pinot Noir was described as having "Layers of tobacco, dark cherry and brambly spice carrying into a long, earthy finish." I caught a hint of something vaguely cherry-like.

I'm not really a wine guy and I probably never will be. Not with so many great beers in the world. But I'm also not the type of non-wine guy who thinks that wine culture is pretentious and full of baloney. While I was unable to name more than one flavor association per wine, every wine I was served at La Crema and at Murphy-Goode was utterly distinct to my palate. I left La Crema feeling pretty certain that if I tasted a flight of wines every day, I might eventually taste most of what the experts said I should.

Our final stop was Hawley, where we arrived after a seven-block slog through now 110-degree heat, which was briefly interrupted by an abrupt plunge into a boutique, where Nataki bought a dress to wear at dinner. What the Hawley wines lacked in appeal, the tasting room made up for in atmosphere. A hired man was playing piano at the far end of the room. I noticed he was rather good. Minutes later I found out he was even better on the guitar. Feeling expansive, I dragged the poor fellow into conversation. His name was Randy. I praised his playing, bought one of his CDs, and casually let slip that my wife could carry a tune. Before I knew it, Nataki was belting out "Summertime" to Randy's six-string accompaniment. The staff watched us blandly from behind the bar as though this kind of stuff happened every day.

To Your Health

The first wines were drunk by people in the region of modern Iran and Armenia around 6000 B.C.E., when it was discovered that grapes or grape juice stored in pottery for a long time fermented. Ancient archaeological references to wine suggest that its early drinkers appreciated its sophistication and variety no less than today's connoisseurs do.

Like coffee and chocolate, wine was used in religious rituals before it became a social drink. It was also used medicinally.

"Drink no longer water, but use a little wine for thy stomach's sake and thine infirmities," the Apostle Paul advised his disciple Timothy. Before that, Hippocrates prescribed wine to treat fever, diarrhea, and pain.

Modern medical science has created a new list of wine's health benefits. Evidence that alcohol in moderation protects against heart disease, the current leading cause of death, was first discovered in the 1930s. Subsequent research demonstrated that alcohol achieves this effect by increasing blood levels of HDL cholesterol and by reducing fibrinogen, a coagulant that gets trapped in arterial plaques. There are some people who prefer to believe that wine alone among alcoholic beverages is good for the heart and that antioxidants, not alcohol itself, are the source of its benefits. In fact, all beverages containing alcohol are more or less equally salutary in this regard. It's true, though, that wine, particularly red wine, contains antioxidants, and these chemicals offer other health benefits. Resveratrol, for example, is a red-wine antioxidant that has been linked to slower aging in mice.

Epidemiological studies have shown that moderate drinking reduces the risk of diabetes and also lowers markers of systemic inflammation, which underlies many chronic diseases. Moderate drinkers, like coffee fiends, even live longer than abstainers. The University of Cambridge Medical Research Council included moderate alcohol consumption on a selective list of four behaviors that increase lifespan. The other three were not smoking, exercising regularly, and eating five servings of fruits and vegetables per day. And yet, like coffee and chocolate, alcohol remains proscribed or severely restricted in some healthy-diet cults, including the Maker's Diet and some low-carb diets.

Pleasurably Healthful
The parallels among wine, coffee, and chocolate are striking. All three are special treats that humans created through the

processing of natural offerings that, while beneficial to health, are consumed primarily for pleasure and enjoyment. What's most interesting about coffee, chocolate, and wine is that the pleasure they give us is directly connected to some of their beneficial health effects.

Many lovers of these special treats have observed that their unique flavors cultivate a refined palate, and in so doing discourage overindulgence. Lucy Gustafson told me, "I made these recipes so that one piece is really all you need." She succeeded. In my estimation, one good truffle is worth a whole box of Oreos.

Thomas Jefferson made a similar point about wine. "No nation is drunken where wine is cheap," he wrote. The wine culture generally disdains drinking to intoxication. While there are many "winos" in the world, oenophiles believe that if you drink to get buzzed, you can't really be very serious about drinking for the sensory experience.

Science supports this perspective, having shown that people who eat to savor food and who have the tasting skills to do it well are less prone to overeat than are cruder tasters. The more you get out of each bite, the fewer bites you take.

In a 2002 study, Beverly Tepper, a professor of food science at Rutgers University, tested the taste sensitivity of eighty-six women. She categorized some as "non-tasters," others as "medium tasters," and the rest as "super tasters." On average, the super tasters weighed 20 percent less than the non-tasters.

While taste sensitivity is largely inborn, with practice anyone's palate can become more sophisticated. The French, who are 50 percent less likely than Americans to be obese—despite eating more chocolate—are better tasters than Americans are for cultural reasons, not genetic ones (although, sadly, this is changing as American food becomes increasingly popular among the French).

The pleasure we get from coffee, chocolate, and wine does more than discourage overindulgence. It is also intrinsically healthy.

Many forms of pleasure and enjoyment, including laughing with friends, listening to music, and savoring good food and drinks, enhance physical health. Japanese researchers found that in a population of 80,000 adults, those who reported experiencing the least pleasure and enjoyment in life were almost two times more likely to die of a heart attack or stroke over a twelve-year period than were those who experienced the most pleasure and enjoyment. Makes you think.

The Pleasure-or-Health Myth

The healthy-diet cults came about as a reaction against the cult of pleasure eating, particularly its bad health effects. In a strange way this has made them inheritors of ascetic traditions that mistrusted the bliss aroused by coffee, chocolate, and wine. To win new followers, the healthy-diet cults must continually overcome people's all-too-easily indulged desire to eat strictly for pleasure. Therefore, the healthy-diet cults are by and large dismissive of the eating experience. Enjoyment is a distraction. The cults are focused almost entirely on the physical health effects of foods.

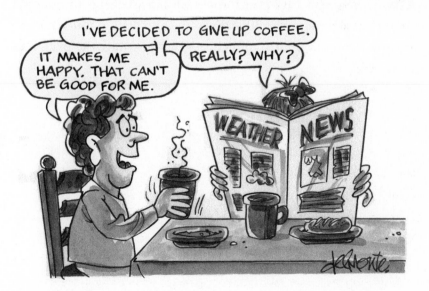

Coffee, chocolate, and wine expose the foolishness of this Puritanism. All three enhance physical health both directly and indirectly, through the enjoyment and pleasure they confer. These gifts also challenge the idea that, when eating for physical health and eating for pleasure are not compatible, it is always right to choose the first. While overindulging in coffee or chocolate or wine is not physically healthy, a person who allows himself to do such things once in a while is likely to be happier, if not physically healthier, than one who does not.

But what is happiness if not spiritual health? And is not the spirit as important as the body? If we grant that total health encompasses both physical and spiritual health, then eating four chocolate truffles and drinking a bottle of wine could be the healthiest thing you do on a given day.

Personally, I'm not quite prepared to follow Lucy Gustafson's choice to skid into her coffin sideways in a worn-out body. A *mostly* healthy life is the life I prefer. But I would rather be Lucy than a diet-cult saint. There have been many days in my life when everything I ate and did was physically healthy. I don't remember most of those days. But I'll never forget that hot weekend in Sonoma when I drank too much coffee and wine and ate too much chocolate (not to mention meat and cheese) with my favorite person in the world.

10

Sugar Water

On a hot August day in 1965, University of Florida assistant football coach Dewayne Douglas visited the office of assistant medical professor Robert Cade, a kidney specialist, and asked the following question:

"Why don't our players pee after games?"

Cade did not know the answer, but he supposed it had something to do with sweat. Perhaps the body responded to sweat-induced dehydration by shutting down urine production to conserve body fluid.

This explanation made sense to Douglas, who told Cade that he had lost as much as eighteen pounds during games in his playing career, which had included a stint with the New York Giants. Cade was astounded. Eighteen pounds! His curiosity piqued, the professor began to investigate the phenomenon of exercise-induced dehydration. He knew that perspiration was a vital cooling mechanism for the body, but he couldn't help but wonder if its benefits came at a cost. Could the body lose so much water during exercise in the heat that it no longer had enough left to cool itself adequately?

Cade's early investigations suggested that it might. Measurements taken on University of Florida football players during hot practices in September 1965 revealed that the longer they remained active, the more weight they lost, the more their blood volume decreased, the hotter they became, and the lower their blood-sugar levels fell. The players were always exhausted at the end of these practices. Cade's measurements seemed to explain why.

Back then, it was not customary for athletes to drink during exercise. Most coaches actively discouraged it, believing that it caused cramps and that an athlete who made a habit of indulging his thirst in the middle of training and competition risked becoming mentally soft. Even long-distance runners seldom interrupted the rhythm of their breathing for a sip of water. Marathons in the 1960s had no official water stations. Most participants ran the full 26.2 miles without drinking anything.

Cade's research led him to think that perhaps athletes *should* drink during activity. But not just water. Cade whipped up a concoction that included water as its base but also contained salt to replace the minerals lost in sweat and sugar to keep blood-sugar levels from dipping. Cade asked the Gators' head football coach, Ray Graves, for permission to test it on his team. Wary of gimmicks, Graves allowed the doctor to give the funny-tasting mix to the freshman team in a scrimmage against the B team. The results were stunning. Fueled by Cade's elixir, the lowly freshmen trounced the more experienced B team, scoring several touchdowns in the fourth quarter, when the younger players seemed impervious to the fatigue that had slowed their opponents to a crawl. No longer skeptical, Graves gave Cade the go-ahead to supply the varsity squad with his magical punch. The Florida Gators soon developed a reputation as a dominant second-half team, and the secret to their endurance became known as Gatorade.

The legend of Gatorade spread throughout the Southeastern Conference. Knock-off brews appeared on the sideline benches of the Florida State Seminoles, the Georgia Bulldogs, and other teams. By 1967, Cade recognized that there was a market for his bottled sweat. He trademarked the name that had been popularly assigned to it and sold the formula to Stokely-Van Camp, Inc., whose most recognizable product at the time was canned pork and beans. Gatorade's new owner (and patent holder) faced a twofold challenge in marketing the product to the broad sporting public. First, it had to convince athletes that dehydration during physical activity was a problem that should be prevented. Second, it had to convince the same market that Gatorade was better than water for rehydration. The company decided it needed scientific studies proving these two points. And it got them.

The first study was led by Robert Cade himself. He recruited six volunteers and had them run and walk for seven miles on a treadmill in a hot environment. Each subject was required to complete the task three times on separate occasions, drinking Gatorade in one trial, plain water in another, and nothing in a third. (The actual order of the trials was randomized.) Cade observed that when the subjects drank nothing and became more dehydrated, their core body temperature increased faster. This finding seemed to establish that dehydration was indeed a problem—specifically, a risk factor for overheating during physical activity. Cade also found that, on average, the subjects completed the seven-mile test 3 percent faster with Gatorade than with plain water or nothing. This finding seemed to establish that Gatorade was a better choice than plain water for hydration.

The publication of these findings in 1972 incited a frenzy of new research. Dehydration, rehydration, body temperature regulation, and the effects of fluid, mineral, and sugar consumption on exercise performance became the hottest research topics in all of sports science. The studies piled up like cement blocks to build a seemingly unshakable fortress of scientific doctrine supporting the use of Gatorade (and the inevitable avalanche of copycat products) during exercise.

The fully formed "Gatorade doctrine" that emerged from this research had five basic tenets:

1. Progressive dehydration during exercise causes blood volume to decline. Less blood delivers less oxygen to the muscles. Oxygen-starved muscles fatigue faster. A lowered volume of blood also produces less sweat to transfer excess body heat to the atmosphere.

2. Unchecked dehydration during prolonged exercise in the heat is potentially dangerous because it allows the core body temperature to increase to health-threatening levels.

3. To minimize the effects of dehydration on performance and on the risk of heatstroke, athletes and exercisers need to drink as much as possible.

4. Thirst is not a trustworthy guide to drinking, as athletes who drink by thirst still become dehydrated.

5. Sports drinks such as Gatorade are preferable to water because their mineral content helps maintain normal electrolyte concentrations in intercellular fluids and because their sugars provide an extra energy source that boosts performance.

The Gatorade doctrine quickly spread from the sports science academy—where it was universally accepted—to coaches, trainers, nutritionists, athletes, sports media professionals, and ultimately the popular media. The driving force of the diffusion was Gatorade itself, which was bought by the Quaker Oats Company in 1983. Quaker perfected the system of science-based marketing that it inherited from Stokely. In 1988 the company created the Gatorade Sports Science Institute, whose mission was to "share current information and expand knowledge on sports nutrition and exercise science that enhances the performance and well-being of athletes." Not long after its foundation, the GSSI became a "Platinum Level" sponsor of the American College of Sports Medicine, the world's largest and most respected exercise science institution.

In 1996, the ACSM published a position statement on exercise and fluid replacement, which asserted that athletes should "attempt to consume fluids at a rate sufficient to replace all the water lost through sweating (i.e., body weight loss), or consume the maximal amount that can be tolerated."

In 1999, Bob Glover and Shelly Lyn-Lawrence cited this position statement in *The Competitive Runner's Handbook*, a popular training guide for runners. "If you wait until you are thirsty to drink, it may be too late," they warned. Runners took heed. One study reported that the average participant in the Houston Marathon between 2000 and 2003 drank twenty cups of water and Gatorade during the event. Many runners quaffed so much of the lemon-lime potion that they actually *gained weight* while running 26.2 miles.

Gatorade's science-based marketing system was so successful that it not only changed the behavior of athletes (in all sports, not just running), but it also changed how the public thought about dehydration. Before Gatorade, a person was either thirsty or not thirsty. Thirst was no big deal—drinking took care of it. If you were very thirsty and there was nothing available to drink—well, that might eventually become a problem. But as Gatorade gained influence, dehydration came to be seen as a sort of disease that was distinct from thirst. Athletes were convinced that they couldn't trust their thirst to tell them when to drink, as though this wasn't like believing a person couldn't trust his bowels to tell him when to visit the bathroom.

The conditions were set for the emergence of a hydration-based diet cult. In 1992, an Iranian emigrant to the United States named Fereydoon Batmanghelidj published a book titled *Your Body's Many Cries for Water*, and the cult was born. Dr. Batmanghelidj taught that dehydration either caused or contributed to heart disease, diabetes, depression, colitis, attention deficit disorder, various cancers, arthritis, fibromyalgia and other autoimmune diseases, asthma, migraine, AIDS, allergies, and a host of other health problems. Although "Batman" (as his followers called him) prescribed water (not sports drinks) to prevent and treat all of these disorders, his concepts were borrowed from the Gatorade doctrine. Gatorade's "voluntary dehydration" during physical activity became Batman's "unintentional chronic dehydration." Batman also followed Gatorade's lead in claiming that the thirst mechanism was unreliable.

Your Body's Many Cries for Water was very successful, finding a home among other alarmist nutrition titles such as *Alkalinize or Die* in health-food stores across the country. A third edition of the book was released in 2008, four years after Batmanghelidj died. According to one source, worldwide sales of all editions have topped 350,000 copies.

The success of the book caught the attention of Stephen Barrett, founder of quackwatch.com, who published an expose on Batmanghelidj. Barrett exhaustively checked out Batman's claims and found no scientific evidence to support any of them—except the claim that water was good for heartburn. Barrett also checked into Batmanghelidj's claims about his background in research and treatment and discovered that most of them were fictional.

No one in the medical establishment gave credence to Ferey-doon Batmanghelidj's half-baked notions. He had taken the whole hydration thing too far. But what the medical establish-ment did not recognize was that the Gatorade doctrine itself, which the medical establishment backed, had already taken the whole hydration thing too far. Fortunately, science is self-correcting. While entire fields of science can remain blind to false assumptions for some time, the truth always worms its way out eventually. The Gatorade doctrine was a theoretical house of cards standing atop a flimsy foundation of wishful thinking that was destined to crumple, and crumple it did, soon after Batman's overreach.

The tipping point came on April 15, 2002, when Cynthia Lucero, a twenty-eight-year-old clinical psychologist, died after collapsing while running the Boston Marathon. The cause of her death was hyponatremia, or "water intoxication." Following the advice she had so often heard to "drink as much as possible" while running, she did just that. The combination of excessive fluid intake and a perhaps genetically rooted inability to excrete this excess as urine while running, as most people can, caused the sodium concentration of her blood to fall dangerously low. Her body lost control of its compartmental fluid balance and her brain began to swell. The pressure created by this swelling caused her to fall into a coma and ultimately killed her.

Timothy Noakes, an exercise physiologist at the University of Cape Town, South Africa, had been warning the world about the dangers of hyponatremia caused by overhydration during exercise for years before the tragic day. Noakes was one of the few true skeptics in his field, one who assumed that every accepted theory was false until he was personally convinced otherwise. His method was to probe deep into the roots of an established scientific model or explanation to determine whether the research actually supported the conclusion that had been drawn from it. In the 1980s, Noakes returned to the foundational science of the Gatorade doctrine and discovered it did not support the five core tenets.

The cornerstone of the Gatorade doctrine was a study that preceded Robert Cade's first Gatorade study. Authored by a pair of Noakes's compatriots, Cyril Wyndham and Nic Strydom, and published in the *South African Medical Journal* in 1969, it bore the alarming title "The Danger of an Inadequate Water Intake during Marathon Running." Wyndham and Strydom had weighed a number of runners before and after they competed in a couple of twenty-mile races to determine how much water weight they lost and thus how dehydrated the runners became. Core-body-temperature measurements (nothing like a thermometer up your rear after a hard run!) were taken at the end of each race. Turned out the runners who became the most dehydrated during the races were also the hottest. Wyndham and Strydom concluded that dehydration caused the core body temperature to increase during exercise.

The interest of these two men in heat stress came from their work as scientists for the mining industry, where heatstroke was a common hazard. Heatstroke is a potentially fatal condition that occurs when the core body temperature reaches 104 degrees, essentially cooking the vital organs. The hottest runners in Wyndham and Strydom's study were just below that threshold. The trend lines indicated that if the runners had run just a little farther, or drunk a little less (for they had drunk some water during the race), or if the weather had been a little warmer, a major medical emergency might have occurred. Wyndham and Strydom recommended that runners consume approximately thirty ounces of fluid per hour to prevent heatstroke. Later research would reveal that this is more than almost any runner ever drinks voluntarily—hence the notion that thirst is unreliable.

When Tim Noakes looked at this study, he spotted an obvious error. The hottest and the most dehydrated subjects at the end of the two races Wyndham and Strydom had observed were also the two *winners*. The reason the body heats up during exercise is that working muscles generate heat. The harder they work, the more heat they generate. As exercise intensity increases, the sweat rate—hence too the rate of body fluid loss—also increases as the body tries to prevent heat from pooling at its core. Given all of this, it seemed perfectly evident to Noakes that the most dehydrated runners in the Wyndham and Strydom study had not become hotter because they had become more dehydrated. Rather, they had become hotter and more dehydrated simply because they had run faster.

Intensity of exercise, Noakes recognized, was the true cause of core-body-temperature increase. Drinking vast quantities of fluid during exercise therefore was not the best way to prevent overheating: *slowing down* was the best way to prevent overheating. This would explain why all runners—even those capable of winning races—are compelled to run slower in hot weather. Newer research has revealed that a brain-based protective mechanism prevents athletes from exercising themselves to death in the heat by reducing muscle activation, and this is why heat illness is rare even in the hottest endurance competitions. No amount of extra drinking will allow a runner to match his cool-weather pace on a hot day.

Noakes did not come down completely against fluid intake during exercise. The literature did show convincingly that drinking caused a slight reduction in the rate of body-temperature increase. This in turn might allow an athlete to go a little faster at his maximum safe body temperature. It was also clear from the research that the sugar content of sports drinks was a significant performance enhancer.

But was it really necessary to drink as much as possible to get these benefits? Noakes suspected it was not, and in 2000 he tested the suspicion. He recruited eight male distance runners to run for two hours, as fast as they could for the final thirty minutes, on a treadmill inside a seventy-seven-degree room—not once but three times. The subjects were given a sports drink to consume in all three trials, but at different rates. In one trial they were allowed to drink according to their thirst. In another they were given a fixed amount of the sports drink that was less than the amount they drank by thirst. In the remaining trial the subjects were forced to drink at a rate that exceeded their preferred rate but was in line with Gatorade doctrine. Noakes found no difference in core body temperature or performance among the three trials.

What's more, in the forced-drinking trial, two of the eight subjects quit with severe nausea. This finding confirmed a footnote from the earliest Gatorade studies, which reported that drinking even slightly more than thirst dictated while running tended to cause gastrointestinal distress. Of course, this was precisely why long-distance runners drank so little before Gatorade came around. One of the subjects in Robert Cade's original Gatorade validation study was Amby Burfoot, winner of the 1968 Boston Marathon, who later became the editor of *Runner's World*. Burfoot confessed to Noakes that guzzling Gatorade at a forced rate had tied his stomach in knots, and afterward he'd gone right back to drinking nothing during marathons.

Noakes subsequently discovered that on top of everything else, drinking as much as possible during exercise created a risk for hyponatremia in some people. Since then, he has urged athletes to drink by thirst in training and competition. This new model of exercise hydration has been much slower to catch on than was the billion-dollar Gatorade doctrine that it aims to overturn.

In the spring of 2012, I ran the Los Angeles Marathon. Before the start, an announcer kept up a steady chatter over a PA system. His monologue included a brief lecture about the dangers of dehydration, culminating in an earnest reminder to "drink early, drink often, drink as much as you can."

Give Me Some Sugar

A little more than a year before I was advised to overhydrate at the LA Marathon, I had dinner with husband-and-wife professional runners Adam and Kara Goucher at a P. F. Chang's in Portland, Oregon. Midway through the meal, Kara brought up a subject she had obviously been planning to introduce.

"Can I ask you a question?" she said.

"You just did," I said.

Ignoring my corny joke, Kara told me that she had just acquired a new nutrition sponsor, Nutrilite, a division of multi-level marketing giant Amway. One of the company's products was ROC_2O, a sports drink that Kara was now expected to use during races, starting with the Boston Marathon, which was just three months away. But a nutritionist Kara knew casually had told her the product was "garbage" and warned her that if she used it at Boston she would probably get sick to her stomach and fail to finish the race.

These words sent Kara into a panic. While she was not contractually obligated to use ROC_2O in races, it would be awkward if she didn't. But if this nutritionist was right and it really would hurt her performance, there was no way she could risk it. She wanted a second opinion.

"Do you mind checking it out and letting me know what you think?" she asked.

I told her I would. When I did, I discovered that ROC_2O was almost identical to Gatorade. Like Gatorade, the Nutrilite product was isotonic, which means its concentration of dissolved particles was equal to that of human body fluids. The carbohydrate concentration of ROC_2O also matched that of Gatorade, at 6 percent. The specific carbohydrates in ROC_2O were sucrose, fructose, and maltodextrin. Gatorade contains sucrose, fructose, and glucose.

These last three items are sugars. Maltodextrin is not a sugar technically, but it behaves like one. Gatorade is often criticized for its high sugar content. The nutritionist who labeled ROC_2O "garbage" had its sugar content in mind.

While most nutrition scientists agree that a moderate amount of sugar in the diet is completely harmless, the average American today gets 13 percent of his daily calories from added sugars, and that's not harmless. People have a hard time making the simple distinction between a food or nutrient that we eat too much of and a food or nutrient that is inherently toxic and should never be eaten. Predictably, an anti-sugar diet cult has emerged in recent years. Members of this cult believe that sugar is bad in all amounts and contexts, including in sports drinks intended strictly for use during prolonged exercise. It doesn't matter that literally hundreds of studies have shown it improves performance. *Sugar is BAD!*

There aren't many respectable nutrition scientists in the anti-sugar-diet cult, but in 2012 it bagged a big one: Timothy Noakes— the same Tim Noakes who had previously called attention to the problem of overhydration in endurance sports. Out of nowhere Noakes went public with a new diet that took anti-sugar vehemence to a new level. The Noakes diet forbids all refined sugars, all grains, and even most kinds of fruit. I know and respect Tim Noakes and I was rather surprised to learn that he had found religion in this way. His few public statements about the origin of his awakening suggest it happened for deeply personal reasons, and not coincidentally at the age at which Noakes's father developed diabetes, which ultimately killed him. The intellect is prone to panic when forced to confront its extinguishment. The famously atheistic philosopher David Hume's deathbed conversion to Christianity comes to mind as another example of the phenomenon. In any case, Noakes's road to Damascus moment goes to show that no one is too smart or knowledgeable to join—or start—a diet cult.

Noakes spreads his new gospel mainly—and very actively— through his Twitter account, which is a must-follow if you're interested in knowing how the most frothing-mouthed diet cult zealots communicate when alone together. There have been some dramatic moments, such as when Noakes apologized to all of the athletes "whose diabetes [he] may have caused" by encouraging them to use sports drinks in his book, *Lore of Running*.

He needn't be so hard on himself. Epidemiological research has demonstrated that there is no independent link between the amount of sugar a person consumes and the risk of diabetes. The American Diabetes Association includes "Eating too much sugar causes diabetes" on its list of the top diabetes myths.

There is evidence, however, that consuming large amounts of *particular forms of sugar*—especially sugar-sweetened beverages—increases the risk of becoming overweight and developing diabetes and heart disease. The biology is complex and not yet fully understood. The bottom line is that there is some justification for the bad reputation that sugar has acquired. One study found that women who consumed one or more sugary drinks per day were 83 percent more likely to become diabetic than were women who drank less than one a month.

Sports drinks are technically sugar-sweetened beverages. It's easy to lump them in with the others, and many nutrition scientists do. In a 2010 review, Frank Hu, a nutritional epidemiologist at Harvard University, pointed a finger at "the full spectrum of soft drinks, carbonated soft drinks, fruitades, fruit drinks, *sports drinks*, energy and vitamin water drinks, sweetened iced tea, cordial, squashes, and lemonade" (my emphasis).

Anyone can recognize that there is a difference between drinking a sports drink while reclining on a La-Z-Boy in front of the television and drinking a sports drink while running a marathon. Few competitive athletes are concerned that using sports drinks in training and competition will make them diabetic. But many are now concerned that the sugar in sports drinks could sabotage their performance by triggering a massive "insulin spike" that in turn will cause a "blood-sugar crash" and exhaustion.

If ingesting sugar during exercise actually did this, then sports drinks would not enhance endurance performance by 2 to 4 percent as they have repeatedly been shown to do. Far from causing a blood-sugar crash during exercise, sugar *prevents* it. During exercise, the pancreas releases glucagon, a hormone that breaks down liver glycogen and shuttles it into the blood stream so that blood-glucose levels remain stable even though thirsty active muscles are rapidly pulling glucose out of the bloodstream. Thanks to glucagon, blood-glucose levels begin to drop only when exercise continues so long that the liver itself runs out of glycogen. Rather than hastening this catastrophe, using a sports drink significantly delays it because the sugars in the product have a sparing effect on liver glycogen.

Simply stated, sugar is the primary reason that sports drinks like Gatorade enhance athletic performance. Their hydrating effect is secondary. That is why the subjects in Robert Cade's first Gatorade study completed the seven-mile walk-run test faster with Gatorade than with plain water. Many subsequent studies have confirmed that water plus sugar boosts exercise performance more than plain water.

Nowadays, though, anti-sugar prejudice has left many athletes unable to wrap their heads around the idea that sugar could ever be beneficial in any context. Even some entrepreneurs in the sports nutrition market can't quite grasp it, so they've developed low-sugar sports drinks that either contain small amounts of sugar or use complex carbohydrates instead of sugars. The makers of these products proudly boast of how much less sugar they contain than Gatorade does, which is ironic, because it is this very thing that makes these products decidedly *less* effective than Gatorade and its imitators.

The problem with low-sugar sports drinks is that they simply don't provide enough energy to the muscles. The optimal rate of carbohydrate intake during exercise is roughly sixty grams per hour. An athlete who takes in half that amount gets 25 percent less benefit. A typical low-calorie sports drink such as Vitamin Water contains roughly half as much sugar as a conventional sports drink like Gatorade. It is less effective for precisely this reason. To suggest that one sports drink is better than another because it contains only half as much sugar is the logical equivalent of suggesting that one commuter car is better than another because it gets half the gas mileage.

Sports drinks that substitute starches for sugars fall short in a similar way. While starchy sports drinks typically provide as much energy as sugary sports drinks, they provide it in a form that is absorbed and metabolized much more slowly. The makers of starchy sports drinks tout the slow action of their products as a benefit. They say their products provide "long-lasting energy" instead of causing a quick energy spike followed by a crash. We have already seen that sports drinks do not cause, but rather delay, a blood-sugar crash during exercise. The problem with slow-acting carbohydrates is that during intense exercise, the muscles burn carbs faster than the body can absorb them. So when a starchy sports drink is consumed, the muscles essentially sit around waiting for those carbs to arrive, whereas the glucose derived from a sugary sports drink reaches the muscles more quickly. The muscles therefore are able to work harder and preserve more of their glycogen supplies for later use. "Lasting energy" sounds good, and at rest it is good, but during exercise the muscles need *fast energy*, and there's no faster energy source than sugar. Sports drinks that provide lasting energy provide *slow energy* and, effectively, *less energy*.

A number of years ago, a new sports drink called G-Push was brought to market with much fanfare. Like many sports drinks that had come along before it and many others that have come along after it, G-Push was hyped as superior to conventional sports drinks such as Gatorade because it was formulated to provide sustained energy. G-Push contained a carbohydrate called galactose, which is technically a simple sugar but is a low-glycemic (i.e., slow) sugar because it has to be processed by the liver before entering the bloodstream, unlike other sugars, such as sucrose, which is broken down to glucose in the stomach and intestine.

In 2009, a team of researchers at New Zealand's Massey University pitted a galactose sports drink against a conventional glucose-fructose sports drink in a cycling performance test. The conventional sports drink blew the doors off the galactose drink formulated to provide "lasting energy." When the cyclists were given the glucose-fructose drink, they were able to complete the time trial in a little more than thirty-three minutes. When they were given the galactose drink, the ride took nearly thirty-eight minutes. The slower-acting sugar just couldn't supply energy fast enough to satisfy the glucose-guzzling active muscles.

There are some anti-sugar zealots who concede that sugary sports drinks perform better than low-sugar and starchy sports drinks. But they've got to find *something* wrong with them, so they blame sugar for causing gastrointestinal distress during exercise. This was essentially the basis of the warning given to Kara Goucher by the nutritionist who called ROC_2O garbage.

It's just more wishful thinking. There is no evidence that low-sugar or starchy sports drinks are less likely to cause nausea and bloating during exercise than are conventional sports drinks. The average rate of GI distress in marathons is 4 percent. The rate of conventional sports-drink use in marathons is closer to 100 percent. What's more, a little stomach discomfort may be a price worth paying in the quest for maximum performance. In Ironman triathlons, participants who consume more carbs finish the race faster even though they suffer more GI symptoms.

After I checked out ROC_2O, I told Kara Goucher that, in my opinion, it was fine—basically Gatorade with a few cosmetic differences. She used it during the Boston Marathon and ran her best time ever, in the process becoming the fourth-fastest American female marathoner in history. And for the first time in any marathon, she suffered no gastrointestinal problems.

The Myth of Absolutes

Diet cults like to make rules that are absolutist in nature. Such rules rest on the belief that the healthiness or unhealthiness of different foods and nutrients is intrinsic to them and does not vary by context. Although each diet cult has its own set of rules, there is universal agreement among the healthy-diet cults that "good" nutrition is always good, no matter when or how it is consumed, and that "bad" nutrition is bad in any context. So pervasive is this message that even people who don't belong to any particular diet cult are prone to fall for such black-and-white thinking about food and nutrients, and perhaps suffer the consequences.

Water has almost always and everywhere been considered good. Belief in the absolute context-free goodness of water made athletes and, somewhat later, society at large susceptible to the Gatorade doctrine, which created an irrational fear of dehydration and encouraged occasionally lethal overhydration.

Sugar was once deemed good but is now judged bad. Belief in the pure badness of sugar has caused many athletes to miss out on an easy opportunity to perform better. And in at least one instance, it has caused an intelligent and well-meaning person with a doctoral degree in nutrition to give potentially career-damaging advice to a world-class athlete whose livelihood depended on squeezing the last 1 percent out of her potential. It makes you want to slap your forehead.

11

Starve or Die

n 2004, the illusionist and endurance artist David Blaine fasted for forty-four days inside a small glass box that was suspended over the River Thames in London. When he was released from his self-imposed captivity, the thirty-year-old Brooklyn native weighed 154 pounds, down fifty-five pounds from his starting weight. He had palpitations of the heart and open sores in his mouth—an early symptom of scurvy. His digestive system had deteriorated to the point where he had to be slowly and carefully reintroduced to nutriments in a hospital setting. An immediate fast-food splurge literally might have killed him. A full medical examination performed in the hospital where Blaine was initially restored to vigor revealed that his liver was functioning abnormally and his hormones were all out of whack.

No sooner had Blaine's feet touched the earth than he dissolved into tears. "This has been one of the most important experiences in my life," he said weakly from the center of a dense throng of admirers and mockers and gawkers and press. "I've learned more in that little box than I have in years. I learned to appreciate all the simple things in life. A smile from a stranger or a loved one. The sunrise. The sunset. Everything that God has given us. And I thank you all so much. I love all of you forever. I love you all! I love you!"

Several days later, looking somewhat less cadaverous, Blaine explained these remarks to an amused Larry King on CNN. "It was just such an emotional moment for me," Blaine said. "At that point, I was living on adrenaline. Everything was rushing through me, and it was sad and beautiful at the same time. To finally be released was just so overwhelming for me."

This was not Blaine's first fast. He had been introduced to fasting as a child in a Jewish household. Observant Jews fast for twenty-four hours on the high holy day of Yom Kippur. But just one day without food was not enough of a challenge for young master Blaine, who had been born with an insatiable hunger (so to speak) to test his ability to withstand prolonged privation and discomfort. So while the rest of the family quit after a single rotation of the planet, little Davy continued for another two days without food, or even water—and then sat in a steam room until he was on the verge of passing out. By the time he was eleven, Blaine had extended his Yom Kippur fast to ten days.

To casual observers, Blaine's circus-like fasting spectacle looked like anything but a spiritual endeavor. They saw nothing more than a performance-art stunt documented and globally disseminated for profit through electronic media. But on closer inspection, the religious origin of Blaine's fasting ability was evident in his London fast. He brought few comforts and distractions into the box with him. Through frosty October nights he slept (or tried to) on a thin camping mattress under an even thinner blanket. His sole luxury was a magic marker. On the glass wall of his enclosure Blaine wrote, "God, faith, will and water." These were the four things he required to endure the test—listed, he told King, in order of importance. Blaine understood before he even entered the box that denying the physical self in such a way was an inherently spiritual experience. Indeed, fasting is and always has been one of mankind's most unobstructed doorways to the realm of spirit.

Closer to God

Not eating for long periods of time when food is readily available is something that most animals never do except in cases of sickness. Only humans fast for non-utilitarian reasons. Scholars believe the phenomenon began as a religious ritual. Most ancient religions observed ritual fasts. In many early cultures, fasting symbolized death and rebirth. Laden with such symbolism, the practice was used in rites of passage and in ceremonies of initiation.

Various Native American peoples incorporated fasting into vision quests, which marked the transition from childhood to adulthood. In a typical ritual the seeker would go off alone into the wilderness for several days, usually fasting the whole time. Other common elements of the vision quest were sleep deprivation, ingestion of hallucinogenic substances such as peyote, and singing. The goal was to experience a vision or dream that communicated a special message from the seeker's guardian spirit, typically some form of animal.

There is, of course, nothing supernatural about the capacity of extreme hunger, sleep deprivation, isolation, and peyote to induce visions. David Blaine experienced distortions of all five senses during his long fast. "There was just a whole heightened sense of everything," he told *Time* magazine. "Taking everything away like that really sharpens colors, tastes, senses, smells, hearing."

Fasting was also used to induce visions in the mystery religions of ancient Greece. The mystery religions were known as such because their practices were clandestine, revealed only to those who passed through sacred initiation rituals that were themselves kept secret. One of the mystery religions that flourished between the fourth and second centuries B.C.E. was the cult of Asclepius, the Greek god of medicine and healing. The sick traveled to temples of Asclepius for healing rituals. They would purify themselves through fasting, ritual baths, and sacrifices before spending a night alone in the temple, where, if all went well, the patient would experience a vision that would reveal his cure.

In some early cultures, religious fasting was exclusive to the priestly class. Among the Evenki people of southern Siberia, fasting was used for thousands of years by shamans to communicate with spirits through visions. (The word "shaman" is Evenki in origin.) Like shamans in other cultures, Evenki shamans were charged with receiving messages from gods and spirits, petitioning those same gods and spirits on behalf of their people, and healing the sick and injured. Much of their work was done in a trance state, and fasting was often used to induce it.

Early cultures believed in the literal reality of the spiritual purification or rebirth that occurred through fasting. Modern anthropologists do not. Instead, they see the rites of passage and initiation ceremonies which included fasting as having served important social functions that benefited the group as a whole. The visions brought on by fasting carried value not just for the one who saw the vision but for the entire culture, nurturing feelings of collective identity and unity.

The function of fasting changed during the so-called Axial Age, which the philosopher Karl Jaspers, who coined the term, placed between 800 and 200 B.C.E., a period when human consciousness achieved new depth and richness, paving the way for the emergence of the major world religions. Within this period, fasting evolved from a means of connecting the group to the celestial realm to become a vehicle for individual connection to the divine. Fasting wasn't so much about purification or symbolic rebirth anymore, but about taming the flesh and controlling the passions to express piety or serve penance.

Among the great prophets of the Axial Age was Confucius, who lived in the fifth and fourth centuries B.C.E. The fourth-century (C.E.) Chinese philosopher Chuang Tzu wrote a dialogue that conveyed the Confucian understanding of fasting. As the story goes, a young man named Yen Hui came to Confucius for help with a personal problem.

"May I ask what to do?" Yen Hui asked.

"You must fast," Confucius said. "I'll tell you why. Is it easy to work from preconceived ideas? Heaven frowns on those who think it is easy."

"My family is poor," Yen Hui said. "I have neither drunk wine nor eaten for many months. Can this be considered fasting?"

"That is the fasting one does for sacrificial ceremonies," Confucius answered, "not the fasting of the mind."

"May I ask what is fasting of the mind?" Yen Hui asked.

"Your will must be one. Do not listen with your ears but with your mind. Do not listen with your mind but with your vital energy. Ears can only hear, mind can only think, but vital energy is empty, receptive to all things. Tao abides in emptiness. Emptiness is the fasting of the mind."

Honestly, I have no clue what Confucius was trying to say here, but it is evident at least that, for him, fasting was much more psychological than it was in the early religions. Like other Axial prophets, Confucius promoted fasting less as a tool for interaction with gods than as a tool for obtaining godly wisdom.

In the biblical Book of Matthew, Jesus completes the most famous fast in history (or in literature, if you prefer). We are told that Jesus was led by "the Spirit" into the wilderness to be tempted by the devil. There he fasted for forty days and forty nights. With typical unintended humor, the scripture states that, at the end of this period, "he was hungry." The tempter then came to him and said, "If you are the Son of God, tell these stones to become bread." But Jesus didn't fall for it.

"It is written," he said: "'Man shall not live on bread alone, but every word that comes from the mouth of God.'"

In this story, the fast is presented as an end in itself, rather than as a means to some other end as in older rituals. For Jesus—and presumably for his followers and for other Jews of his time as well—the purpose in going hungry was not to trigger visions but to give the body an opportunity to gain control over the mind, and then to thwart the coup. The challenge of the fast was to resist the temptation of food and thereby reassert the mind's dominance. Success strengthened the mind and placed the flesh in subjugation to it, which pleased God.

The faithful of all the major religions have used fasting for such spiritual self-improvement ever since this story was written. But some scholars believe that the arrival of the modern age changed the meaning of fasting once again, making it even more temporal and psychological. In our time there are many Jews, Christians, Buddhists, Muslims, and others who have lost their religion to some extent yet continue to fast periodically because they get something useful out of it. According to the sociologist Joseph Tamney, these nominal and lapsed believers have discovered that the training in self-control they get from fasting helps them nego-tiate life's vagaries. They no longer care so much if their sacrifices are pleasing to God. There is an intrinsic benefit of fasting that they enjoy regardless of God's opinion.

In Chapter 5 we saw that self-control—the scientific word for willpower—has important effects on how life turns out for the individual. People with strong self-control are wealthier, healthier, and happier than people with weaker willpower. Experiences that strengthen self-control are rewarding even though they are difficult. This is one of the reasons participation in marathons, triathlons, and other extreme endurance sport events has become so popular, and it may be one of the reasons semi-religious and even irreligious people practice religious or spiritual fasts today.

In 2012, an Indonesian journalist named Abdul Qowi Bastian interviewed people who observed the Ramadan fast despite having formally renounced Islam. One subject, a nineteen-year-old woman, explained, "I'm not fasting for the sake of religion but as a way to practice humility and self-control. These elementary qualities become feats because of the way in which we as a society worship worldly pleasures and material goods. I'm simply diverting my attention from worldly needs to find peace."

In the West, fasting these days is often done in the form of a juice cleanse, which is ostensibly a secular practice. If ancient peoples sought to purify the body through fasting in order to curry the favor of divine beings, many nonreligious people today seek to purify the body for the sake of purifying the body. The typical juice cleanse consists of three or four days of consuming little or nothing besides fresh juices from fruits and vegetables. The specific purpose of juice-fasting is to remove accumulated toxins from the body. Science does not validate this concept. The body contains organs—namely the liver and kidneys—that are designed for detoxification and do the job quite well. Some artificial toxins, such as BPA from plastics, are able to slip through the body's built-in detoxification mechanisms. But there is no evidence that juice-fasting deals with these pollutants any better.

Science's rejection of the purported physical benefits of juice-fasting has done nothing to dampen enthusiasm for the practice in the "natural health" community where it is most popular. Perhaps this is because its real benefits are not physical but spiritual after all. While juice-fasters often report feeling great during and after the experience, that feeling may be nothing more than the same sense of self-control that other fasters enjoy. There is a degree of acknowledgement of juice-fasting's spiritual core in the fact that some of the most popular diet books sold at New Age stores are guides to juice-fasting.

A person may or may not need religion to get by in the modern world. One does, however, need self-control. Although fasting originated as a religious practice, it remains popular in the modern world even among those who have lost their formal religion because it strengthens all-around willpower. Controlled starvation is, in a very fundamental sense, healthy for the mind.

Starve a Fever

Although humans are the only animals that fast when they are healthy and food is available, many animals, including humans, refuse food when they are sick. The first experiences of fasting that our ancestors had were undoubtedly only the semi-voluntary fasts that occurred during bouts of illness. These experiences may have given rise to the idea that fasting was an effective medicine. If a person falls ill, and then doesn't eat, and then returns to health, it is sensible to at least consider the possibility that going without food is partly responsible for the restoration of health.

In the late fifth century B.C.E. Hippocrates, known as the father of medicine, promoted fasting as pharmacon, writing, "Everyone has a physician inside him or her; we just have to help it in its work. The natural healing force within each one of us is the greatest force in getting well. Our food should be our medicine. Our medicine should be our food. But to eat when you are sick is to feed your sickness."

The Hippocratic theory of sickness and health survived for two thousand years. But when scientific medicine emerged in the twentieth century, many of Hippocrates's beliefs started to look crude and silly, including the idea that to eat when you are sick is to feed the sickness. How the heck was that supposed to work?

Yet we've since come full circle. Scientists have lately learned that fasting really does starve certain illnesses.

One of the faults of modern medicine is that it lacks respect for instinct. To underestimate the intelligence of instinct is to set oneself up to look like a fool in due time. We saw this in the preceding chapter in the Gatorade doctrine's dismissal of thirst as a cue to drink, and we see it again here in the dismissal of fasting as a response to sickness. Scientists should have known all along that if many animals fast instinctively when they are sick, there must be a good reason. And we now know that reason—for certain illnesses, anyway.

During a fast, the cells of the body behave like a threatened turtle. When deprived of their accustomed influx of nutrients, the cells panic and scramble inside their shell (so to speak). Their internal metabolism slows to a crawl, and their membranes become less permeable so that things which are normally able to get inside cannot. This lockdown effect of fasting on the cells leaves disease-causing foreign invaders shut out and vulnerable to their own perils. In this way, semi-starvation improves symptoms in diseases as diverse as epilepsy and rheumatoid arthritis. But the most interesting example of the effects of fasting on disease is cancer.

Studies led by Valter Longo, head of the Longevity Institute at the University of Southern California, have demonstrated that fasting combats the growth of several types of cancerous tumors in mice. In one study, fasting slowed the spread of breast cancer, glioma, and human neuroblastoma significantly compared to continued eating. Fasting also extended life in mice with human ovarian cancer and was as effective as chemotherapy in the treatment of breast cancer.

In combination with chemotherapy, fasting is even more powerful. As a cancer treatment, chemotherapy is a double-edged sword because it is toxic to both cancer cells and healthy cells.

The challenge has always been to kill the disease without killing the patient. Fasting makes this tightrope-walk easier by putting normal cells in hibernation mode and leaving cancer cells to face a kind of biochemical lean winter. Longo's research has shown that fasting alters the expression of genes that affect cell growth and metabolism. These changes serve to protect normal cells from the toxic insult of chemotherapy. But fasting has the opposite effect on cancer cells, which are actually sensitized to the chemicals used in the treatment. What makes cancers so deadly is their capacity for lightning-fast growth. To gain this advantage, however, they must sacrifice the ability to survive in what Longo refers to as "extreme environments," such as the hormonal milieu created by fasting.

In one study, Longo and his colleagues injected mice with a particularly aggressive cancer and then fasted some of them for two days while allowing the rest to continue eating before all of the sick rodents were given chemotherapy. Six months later, all of the non-fasted mice were dead, while 40 percent of the fasted mice were still alive.

The next step, naturally, was a series of studies involving human cancer patients. These are just getting under way, but the early results are promising. Patients have reported better tolerance for chemotherapy after fasting.

Hunger Cults

Given the physical and mental health benefits of fasting, and given the natural human propensity to form diet cults, it was inevitable that someone would come along and propose that fasting was the solution to everything—the One True Way to total health. That someone was Bernarr Macfadden, who in the early twentieth century claimed that fasting was the single best thing one could possibly do for one's overall well-being. He wrote that through fasting "a person could exercise unqualified control over virtually all types of disease while revealing a degree of strength and stamina such as would put others to shame." At a time when it was believed that no human could live longer than ten days without food, Macfadden routinely fasted for a week at a time.

Macfadden made a fortune as the head of a publishing empire whose flagship product was a magazine called *Physical Culture*. He also established a number of "healthatoriums" that were intended to function as the churches of a new religion, "cosmotarianism," whose god was health and whose sacraments included fasting. In an article on fasting published in *The Atlantic*, Steve Hendricks wrote of Macfadden, "Thousands of disciples followed his advice . . . and for a while it seemed fasting might spread into the broader national consciousness. But in time Macfaddenism faded from public attention, and fasting with it."

The great spoiler of Macfaddenism's hopes for cosmotarian world conquest was the sheer unpleasantness of the fasting experience. To the average person, extreme hunger is about as enjoyable as a day-long cold shower. Macfadden may have overlooked this fly in the ointment in his zealotry. He may also have overhyped the benefits of fasting.

Yet there is one serious health condition that fasting—in principle—treats more effectively than any other medicine: fatness. When he launched *Physical Culture* in 1899, Macfadden could not have known that obesity would one day become his country's greatest public-health concern. And when he died in 1955, he was sadly unaware that fasting was on the brink of a comeback—or at least a vindication.

In Chapter 2, I described the traditional diet of the inhabitants of the island of Crete, which was popularized as the Mediterranean Diet after the American epidemiologist Leland Allbaugh visited the island in 1948 and discovered that its people had the lowest incidence of heart disease of any population on earth. The cardiovascular health of the Cretans was reflexively attributed to the food they ate: lots of fresh fruits and vegetables, nuts, a little seafood, a little meat, and loads of olive oil. But later researchers suspected—and eventually proved—that *not eating* these same foods deserved almost as much credit.

A majority of Cretans belong to the Greek Orthodox Church. If there's one thing that distinguishes this church from other Christian denominations, it's fasting. Strict followers of Greek Orthodox customs fast 180 days each year. If you emailed a Greek Orthodox friend at random and asked if she was fasting, there would be an almost 50-percent chance that she would respond with a "yes." Not all of the fasts on the Greek Orthodox calendar are water-only fasts—but still.

In the early 2000s scientists at the University of Crete tracked sixty fast-observant Greek Orthodox islanders and sixty non-observant control subjects for one year. At the end of that year, the fasters had significantly lower levels of total cholesterol, "bad" cholesterol, and body fat. Subsequent studies have produced similar results, but the research has not been well publicized. Olive oil sales have shot to the moon since the Mediterranean Diet was first packaged, labeled, and marketed beyond its place of origin. Olive oil is wonderful, but it may not be the secret to the health of the Cretans. Frequently *giving up* olive oil—and a whole lot else—may be the real secret.

Fasting is different from merely eating less as a means to lose weight. Eating less is not as extreme as fasting in the sense that it entails a fractional reduction in caloric intake instead of an absolute cessation of nourishment. But regular dieting is more extreme than fasting in the sense that it has no endpoint, whereas fasting, while certainly hardcore, is by its very nature a short-term thing—unless the fast is undertaken as a method of suicide.

In July 1877, a Minneapolis physician named Henry Tanner used fasting as a method of suicide. This was back in the days when it was believed that a man could survive no longer than ten days without food. Tanner survived forty-one days (bettering Christ by one) and then decided to go on living after all.

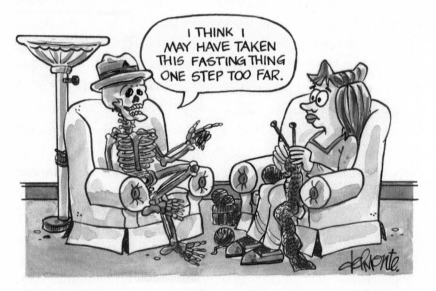

News of Tanner's "miracle" spread far and wide. Three years later, he found himself repeating the feat on stage (setting the bar for David Blaine's later high-production-value performance) in New York City. In forty days, he lost thirty-six pounds. No mainstream weight-loss diet could match those results. But within just eight days of quitting the fast, Tanner had regained all of that weight.

The short-term nature of fasting is its Achilles heel as a tool for weight loss. The human body regains lost fat far more readily— about five times more readily, judging by the mathematics of Tanner's second fast—than it loses it. Anyone who loses a load of blubber through prolonged fasting is bound to gain it all back after the fast ends.

But what about frequent, repetitive, short-term fasting—a "life-style" approach to fasting that basically secularizes the calendar of the observant Greek Orthodox Cretan for the sake of weight management? Intermittent fasting, as it has come to be known, works quite well to improve body composition. In fact, it seems to work at least as well as the usual dieting method of continuous moderate caloric restriction even when fasting is not absolute.

In 2011, a team of English researchers led by Michelle Harvie placed overweight young women on either of two diets for six months. One group was subjected to continuous moderate calorie restriction. The second group ate normally five days per week and ate 75 percent less than normal on the other two days. After six months, members of the intermittent fasting group had lost an average of 7.5 percent more weight than those in the continuous calorie restriction group.

A few efforts have been made to turn intermittent fasting into a popular diet for overweight men and women, but it has only really caught on within the bodybuilding/body sculpting subculture. People in this community had no trouble getting lean and ripped before intermittent fasting came around, but the complex, mathematical nature of the method was a perfect match for the group's ethos. The very popularity of intermittent fasting with the gym-going crowd offers a second inducement for its members to practice it. Whether or not it works any better than good old-fashioned portion control, intermittent fasting has become another way besides protein shakes and supplements (the topic of Chapter 13) for bodybuilders and body sculptors to distinguish themselves from other kinds of eaters.

Long Live the Hungry

In the late nineteenth century, Maurice Gueniot, president of the Paris Medical Academy, developed a reputation for not eating much. When asked why he dined so sparely, Monsieur Gueniot said he believed it was good for his health. Gueniot's peers mostly smiled at the idea—until they all died off. Meanwhile, the abstemious doctor lived to 102.

In 1935, the very year of Gueniot's passing, *The Journal of Nutrition* published a study that suggested a possible link between

Gueniot's gustatory restraint and his longevity. Clive McCay, a biologist at Cornell University, allowed one group of mice to eat as much as they wanted throughout their lives and fed another group of mice 20 percent less (while taking measures to ensure that they got enough vitamins and minerals). On average the mice in the second group lived 16 percent longer. In his report on these findings, McCay refrained from putting forward an explanation for the link between underfeeding and life extension, but it's clear from his language that he suspected it had something to do with the slower growth rate and smaller mature size of the underfed (but not undernourished) mice.

In their efforts to duplicate McCay's discovery, other researchers noted a connection between underfeeding and reduced incidence of specific pathologies, especially malignant tumors. This led some to hypothesize that calorie restriction prolonged life not by slowing the aging process but by preventing disease—cancer in particular. However, subsequent research revealed that, while calorie restriction did indeed thwart some tumors, it extended life primarily by slowing the aging process. But the question of how remained unanswered.

The leading theory for some time was that calorie restriction slowed aging by reducing the basal metabolic rate. This theory presupposed that aging processes were somehow related to metabolism. There is some evidence of such a link. For example, through the normal processing of blood glucose, some glucose molecules bind to proteins and become destroyers of organ tissues. The immune system produces agents called macrophages that gobble up these destructive glycated proteins and prevent them from doing further harm. But as the body ages, the kidneys produce fewer and less potent macrophages and the ravages of glycation accelerate. It is now known, however, that calorie restriction reduces the basal metabolic rate only transiently. After an initial drop, metabolism rebounds in creatures kept on calorie restriction.

Today there is mounting evidence that calorie restriction in fact slows aging in much the same way that fasting increases the effectiveness of chemotherapy. Body cells perceive underfeeding as a stressor to which they respond by stepping up their natural defenses against assault from free radicals. The evolutionary intent of this response was undoubtedly to help creatures survive famine, but under the right circumstances life extension could be an accidental benefit of the same mechanism.

While some scientists raced to figure out how calorie restriction slowed aging, others worked to determine whether calorie restriction extended the lives of species other than mice. This effort led quickly to the discovery that water fleas, fish, worms, hamsters, rabbits, and yeast cultures also benefited from getting less food.

By the late 1980s there was enough evidence of a general effect of calorie restriction on the lifespan across species that researchers at a pair of institutions decided it was worth their while to invest in long-term studies involving animals much more similar to humans: namely, rhesus monkeys. One study was conducted at the Wisconsin National Primate Research Center and the other at Louisiana State University. In 2009, the first group announced that 80 percent of the monkeys that had been on a calorie-restricted diet since birth were still alive, compared to only half of the well-fed monkeys.

Long before this news broke, some people were already practicing calorie restriction in the hope of living longer. In December 1994, the Calorie Restriction Society was formed at a meeting of the Academy of Anti-Aging Medicine in Las Vegas. Its mission is to "understand and promote the Calorie Restriction (CR) Diet." This diet is only loosely defined, but it basically entails eating a lot less than one would otherwise eat while making sure to avoid malnourishment by basing the diet on nutrient-dense whole foods. The Society provides a set of guiding principles but leaves it up to each adherent of the diet to figure out for himself or herself how to achieve the desired calorie restriction. Many followers of the CR Diet aim to take in roughly 1,500 calories a day. Founding Calorie Restriction Society president Brian Delaney hits this mark by skipping lunch.

Nearly twenty years after the Society was founded, only a few thousand people worldwide follow the CR Diet strictly, mostly men. All of them realize they are rolling the dice. Brian Delaney and his hungry friends may discover the hard way that calorie restriction does not extend human life. Every now and again there comes along a study that has to make longevity dieters wince. In 2012, for example, the organizers of that other monkey study, the one at Louisiana State University, reported that calorie restriction had failed to extend life in their subjects. The key difference was that these monkeys—in both the calorie-restricted and non-restricted cohorts—had been fed a much higher-quality diet than had the monkeys in the Wisconsin study.

Perhaps it doesn't matter. Whereas outliving Maurice Gueniot may be the explicit goal of starting the CR Diet, the true payoff is possibly something far less quantifiable.

"My motivation has changed," Delaney said in one interview. "I am less interested in living [a long time] than I used to be. What I like more is the effects of this diet. I wake up and feel young. Then I think, 'I would like to feel the same way tomorrow. And the following day.' That's what leads to the conclusion that it might not be so horrible to live a really long life. I think for most people, it's a sense of curiosity about how it's going to turn out."

The Myth of Must
The healthy-diet cults are big on musts: you must eat this, you must not eat that. In truth there are very few musts in human nutrition. As we saw in Chapter 6, there are forty-six essential nutrients that we must have in adequate amounts to sustain basic health. Eating fruits and vegetables is probably an additional

must for the attainment of maximum health. Everything else is optional. The supposed musts of any diet cult can be defied in careful ways without any cost in well-being.

Indeed, eating itself is only a qualified must. You can eat one third less than you do now and be just as healthy or maybe healthier. You can stop eating for brief periods under an oncologist's supervision and possibly increase your chances of beating cancer. You can eat nothing at all for a week or more and improve your mental health.

Or not. For, despite what the various cults of fasting would have us believe, fasting too is no more a must than is anything else in human nutrition. You can keep eating as much as you do now and—provided your food choices are good—live as long as the semi-starvationists do. You can body-build or body-sculpt without jumping on the intermittent-fasting bandwagon and become ripped and lean nonetheless. And you can achieve enlightenment without voluntary submission to prolonged hunger.

For that matter, voluntary submission to prolonged hunger offers no guarantee of enlightenment. David Blaine learned this the hard way after his forty-four-day fast above the River Thames. When he came down from the glass box, he thought his life would be changed forever. "But as soon as I was re-fed," he told Larry King, "it's like I forgot everything. All those awakenings I had."

12

Scapegluten

T he University of Virginia's graduating class of 1939 included a lanky young man who bore the mildly unfortunate name of William Crook. He was known by his fellow premed students as a bright and congenial chap whose self-effacing charm masked a formidable will and great ambition. After leaving Charlottesville with his diploma, Crook continued his medical training at the Pennsylvania Hospital and Vanderbilt University and at last completed it at Johns Hopkins. In 1949 he returned to his hometown of Jackson, Tennessee, to set up a practice in pediatric and family medicine. He married local girl Betsy Noe and fathered three daughters by her.

Through his work, Crook developed a special interest in the relationship between allergies and nutrition. In 1979 this interest brought him into contact with C. Orian Truss, an Alabama doctor who believed that many common illnesses were caused by yeast infections. After Truss's example, Crook began to diagnose "candidiasis" (named after the offending yeast, *candida albicans*) in his patients and to treat it with a yeast-free diet. He discovered that a great many of his patients were afflicted with this condition, which was not recognized by the medical establishment, and that most sufferers responded well to proper treatment.

In 1983 Crook authored a book titled *The Yeast Connection*, which alerted the public to the hidden candidiasis epidemic and described its cure. In medicine, it is rather unusual for a doctor to go public with a newly discovered illness and its treatment before that illness has been formally recognized, but Crook felt a sense of urgency, and in any case it was obvious that formal recognition of the candida hypothesis was not soon forthcoming.

Candida albicans is a fungus that is present in the intestinal tract and vagina and a few other parts of the human body. A healthy immune system is able to keep it under control; but when the immune system is weakened, candida can multiply and spread to parts of the body where it does not belong. Crook believed that the agent most often responsible for giving candida a foothold was antibiotics. In his book he explained that antibiotics used to treat viral and bacterial infections killed not only the targeted viruses and bacteria, but also some of the antibodies that kept candida in check. An overgrowth of the yeast often followed.

The medical establishment recognizes vaginal yeast infections and a few other conditions related to yeast overgrowth, including hives and thrush (an infection of the tongue and cheeks). Crook argued that candidiasis also caused fatigue, irritability, pre-menstrual syndrome, digestive disorders, muscle pain, attention deficit disorder, hyperactivity, headache, memory loss, impotence, depression, hypoglycemia, learning disabilities, allergies, chemical sensitivity, and possibly also psoriasis, multiple sclerosis, autism, and arthritis. Crook repeatedly used the phrases "feeling bad all over" and "feeling sick all over" to describe how candidiasis sufferers felt.

Most physicians see a lot of patients who feel bad all over and whose cases resist a definitive diagnosis. Doctors are divided on the origin and nature of this *malaise général*. Some in Crook's day dismissed it as "female neurosis" or hypochondria, diagnoses that persist even now. Others always insist on diagnosing something familiar. Still others are not afraid to throw up their hands and confess ignorance. Crook believed that candidiasis lay underneath nearly every case of general malaise. He wrote, "If a careful check-up doesn't reveal the cause of your symptoms, and your medical history . . . is 'typical,' it's possible or even probable that your health problems are yeast connected."

In *The Yeast Connection,* Crook explained that there was no test that could be used to diagnose candidiasis because even the healthiest people have yeast in their bodies. The strongest evidence that candidiasis was present, he said, was a positive response to treatment. If a patient's symptoms and history indicated the likelihood that the underlying problem was yeast, a marked improvement in symptoms after treatment offered confirmation.

The centerpiece of Crook's treatment was a special diet that was based on the regimen he learned from Dr. Truss. Rule number one was to avoid foods containing yeast. While yeast in food did not cause candidiasis, Crook said, it exacerbated the condition. Sweets of all forms, including soft drinks, were forbidden because sugar fueled the spread of yeast. Crook encouraged patients to avoid fruits for the first three weeks on the diet and then cautiously reintroduce them. He discouraged consumption of "most boxed, canned, processed and packaged foods" because they often contained hidden ingredients that could be problematic. Nuts, seeds, and sprouts were to be treated case by case. Their mold content,

Crook explained, worsened symptoms in some but not all candida sufferers. Alcoholic beverages were totally off limits.

As for what *was* allowed on the candida diet, vegetables were to be eaten in great quantities. The best ones, according to Crook, were asparagus, broccoli, cabbage, cucumbers, peppers, greens, lettuce, okra, beans, and squash. The diet also prescribed "good proteins" such as chicken, lean beef, eggs, salmon, mackerel, and other seafood. Unrefined oils, including linseed, safflower, soy, walnut, and corn, were permitted as well. Grains and starchy vegetables were okay in moderation. Approved beverages were filtered water, coffee, and tea.

The success of *The Yeast Connection* exceeded expectations. Crook's opus became a national bestseller, went through three editions, and ultimately racked up one million copies in sales. A large majority of the book's one million purchasers were women. Crook supposed this gender imbalance reflected the simple fact that more women than men suffered from candidiasis. Skeptics thought it likelier that women were more comfortable with the idea of having a yeast problem and were perhaps also more responsive to the notion of feeling bad all over.

Among the hundreds of thousands of women who followed the candida diet in the 1980s was my mother, Laurie Fitzgerald. Laurie did not herself "feel bad all over" at the time she started the diet, but she was dealing with digestive issues. Her major symptoms were persistent intestinal discomfort and (I have her permission to say this) chronic diarrhea. After a few months of quiet suffering with these annoyances, Laurie made an appointment to see her doctor, who diagnosed irritable bowel syndrome. He explained that the cause of IBS was not known and that treatment was limited to symptom management. Laurie was instructed to take wheat germ or a fiber supplement, to avoid gas-forming foods, and to limit the stress in her life. If these measures didn't help, he would prescribe anti-diarrhea medication.

Not long after she had received her diagnosis, my mother shared it with her friend Elizabeth. No great fan of modern Western medicine, Elizabeth told Laurie that diagnosing IBS was a doctor's way of saying he had no idea what was really wrong. She advised my mother to visit a holistic doctor in Boston whom she (Elizabeth) saw regularly and liked.

By this time, William Crook's book had been out for several months and its influence was spreading. Mainstream medical professionals such as the doctor who had diagnosed IBS in my mother dismissed the notion of a candidiasis epidemic as quackery, but alternative-medicine practitioners embraced it. When Laurie arrived at the office of her friend's naturopath, she was handed a ten-page medical-history questionnaire to fill out. If nothing else, it made her feel that she was being taken seriously, something she did not feel with her regular doctor. After reviewing the form, the naturopath told Laurie that she had candidiasis and recommended Crook's diet along with his book.

Laurie dutifully read the book and started the diet. She stopped eating all foods containing yeast or added sugar, cut out refined grains, and reduced her alcohol consumption from little to none. Taking Crook at his word, my mother came to see yeast in food not as a nutritional villain but rather as something she just couldn't eat. But many others on the diet missed the nuances of Crook's theory and came away with the idea that yeast was an inherently bad thing that *caused* candidiasis pure and simple and should never be eaten by *anyone*. Yeast became a nutritional scapegoat, gleefully demonized, blamed for everything.

When she had been on the candidiasis diet for a few weeks, Laurie and her husband, my father, were invited to dinner at a neighbor's house. Her polite refusal of the wine and sweets she was offered there drew unwanted attention and she was obliged to explain her diet. The husband of the host couple, a chemist who fancied that his expertise extended to all things chemical (i.e., the known universe), laughed in Laurie's face, scorning candidiasis as another make-believe malady cooked up by the alternative-medicine crowd. She shook off the embarrassment and persisted with the diet, seldom cheating as the days turned into weeks and the weeks into months. Despite such discipline, my mom's gastrointestinal symptoms did not improve. But she did lose weight—a happy side effect of the diet's restrictive nature. Having started Crook's regimen at 135 pounds, she slimmed down to 123 pounds. Whatever my father thought of the whole candida thing, he approved of this accidental treatment outcome. So what if she ate a little strangely and caused a stir at dinner parties? She hadn't looked so good since their wedding day!

The more successful *The Yeast Connection* became, the more controversy it stirred up. Crook had few defenders among his peers in mainstream medicine. His more charitable critics chastised him for engaging in unscientific speculation and for doing an end run around proper medical research. His less charitable critics called him a reckless and opportunistic fraud whose encouragement of self-diagnosis and self-treatment of a nonexistent disease was almost certainly harming many people suffering from other, real illnesses.

In the second edition of his book, Crook defended himself against his critics, and in the third edition he parried some more. He pointed out that it was not at all unusual for clinical medical practice to get ahead of scientific understanding, citing the example of James Lind, who prevented scurvy in British sailors in the 1740s by supplying them with limes on long sea voyages. Not until 1929 did the guys back at the laboratory discover why this practice worked. If Lind's "sea wisdom" had not been in use during the intervening two hundred years, generations of sailors would have suffered from scurvy instead of coping marvelously as "limeys."

Crook also brought up the case of Ignace Semelweiss, who in 1845 figured out that the dreaded and often fatal "child-bed fever" could be prevented by doctors *washing their hands* prior to performing pelvic examinations on women in labor. Semmelweiss was fired for putting forward such "unscientific anecdotal observations." A quarter of a century and countless needless deaths later, the guys back at the laboratory vindicated Semmelweiss and common sense.

"In my opinion," Crook wrote, "the role of Candida albicans in making millions of people develop health problems resembles, in many ways, the observations of Lind and Semmelweiss."

Unfortunately for Crook, the last chapter of his story did not resemble those of earlier heroes in the struggle against the tyranny of the hidebound medical-science establishment. In May 2002, six months before Crook's death, German researchers published a comprehensive review of the accumulated research on the candida question, which had become extensive. More than a hundred relevant studies were scrutinized. The authors bluntly concluded that "neither epidemiological nor therapeutic studies provide evidence for the existence of the so-called 'Candida-syndrome' or 'Candida-hypersensitivity-syndrome'."

Three years after this blow was dealt, William Crook was posthumously awarded his own page on quackwatch.com. On it, the website's founder, Stephen Barrett (whom we met in Chapter 10), described several historical cases of patients with nonspecific symptoms such as fatigue and depression who had been diagnosed with candidiasis by alternative medical practitioners, when these patients actually had other, sometime serious conditions such as hepatitis.

"I believe that practitioners who diagnose nonexistent 'yeast problems' should have their licenses revoked," Barrett wrote.

By the time these words were written, they hardly mattered on a practical level. Most of the people who had tried Crook's cure in the 1980s had, like my mother, discovered for themselves that it cured nothing. The public had long since found other nutrients to scapegoat.

Next Victim

In 1991, when the great candida crisis was on the wane, eighteen-month-old Tyler Korn was diagnosed with celiac disease. An auto-immune disorder, celiac disease is characterized by the inability to properly digest gluten, a protein in wheat and related grains. Certain rare genetic abnormalities predispose the immune system to react strangely to gluten exposure, attacking the wall of the small intestine as though it were a virus. The resulting damage compromises the intestine's ability to absorb other nutrients. Symptoms of the disease are notoriously variable, but the classic early symptoms in young children are primarily gastrointestinal: gas, cramping, constipation, diarrhea, oily stools, loss of appetite, and weight loss. Tyler Korn exhibited most of these symptoms.

Back then, celiac disease was rarely diagnosed. Tyler's mother, Danna Korn, had never heard of it. When her child's gastro-enterologist referred her to a hospital dietitian whose job was to explain the gluten-free diet that was and still is the only treatment for celiac disease, the dietitian expressed surprise.

"We don't get many of those," she told Korn.

"Really?" Korn said. "How many have you had?"

"None," the dietitian said.

Although celiac disease is easily neutralized by a gluten-free diet, Danna Korn was deeply upset by her son's diagnosis. She felt that she had failed him somehow. Her first trip to the supermarket with the dietitian's guidelines in hand was like something out of a nightmare. *Everything* had gluten in it! Korn was about ready to give up when she reached the snack-chips aisle and discovered that Fritos were gluten-free. She wept tears of relief.

Buoyed by this small victory, Korn set about learning every-thing she could about celiac disease and gluten-free eating. Before long, she knew as much as any doctor did, so she wrote a book: *Kids with Celiac Disease: A Family Guide to Raising Happy, Healthy Gluten-Free Children*. Korn had no illusions of getting rich off this humble literary foray. Targeting the small market of parents of children diagnosed with celiac disease, it was intended to satisfy a need that had gone unsatisfied precisely because so few shared it.

But a strange thing happened in the decade after Tyler Korn received his diagnosis: the number of celiac sufferers exploded, and it continued to grow rapidly through the following decade. A study by researchers at the Mayo Clinic reported a 56-percent increase in the rate of celiac diagnosis between 2000 and 2010. Over the same period of time, the incidence of non-celiac gluten sensitivity also increased drastically. Gluten-sensitive individuals suffer from many of the same symptoms as persons with celiac disease but lack the underlying genetic predisposition and show no signs of intestinal damage.

As the frequency of these conditions increased, so did awareness of them. And as awareness increased, more and more people with gastrointestinal problems and other complaints put themselves on gluten-free diets in the hope of finding relief. By 2005, the number of people on such diets far exceeded the number of people like Tyler who truly needed to be on them. The food industry took notice. The phrase "gluten-free" began to appear prominently on food packaging. At first it was seen only on products that one might suspect of containing gluten—such as Fritos—but in fact did not. Later, companies slapped the phrase on products that contained no grains of any kind, let alone wheat. Still later, gluten was artificially removed from foods that naturally did contain it so that they, too, could wear the attractive label. By this time, many health-food stores had created special gluten-free sections. By 2012, sales of gluten-free products in the United States had reached 4.2 billion dollars.

Surveys have shown that a majority of the people who buy gluten-free products today have little idea why they do. They just have a vague idea that gluten—whatever the heck it is—is bad.

In 2002, when the gluten-free diet trend was gaining momentum, Danna Korn authored a second book, titled *Wheat-Free, Worry-Free: The Art of Healthy, Happy Gluten-Free Living*. The scope of this book was much broader than that of the first. Korn stopped just short of suggesting that the whole world ought to give up gluten. In the introduction, she wrote, "I'm guessing that you're reading this book because you don't feel well, and you suspect that food may be at the root of your problem. It very well could be, especially if you have any of the following symptoms: fatigue, gastrointestinal distress, headaches, inability to concentrate (i.e., ADD/ADHD), inability to gain or lose weight, infertility, joint pain, moodiness or depression, [or] muscle aches."

If you noticed that this list of symptoms looks a lot like William Crook's catalog of candidiasis symptoms, you're not alone. Korn herself cited candidiasis as one of several conditions often confused with celiac disease. Although her book was published at the same time as the scientific review mentioned above that fully discredited the candidiasis hypothesis, Korn took a neutral position on the subject. "The significance of candidiasis in the story of the healthy gut is the subject of controversy," she stated; "some say its importance is overrated, and others say it's key." Korn neglected to say that the "some" who rejected the candida hypothesis included every single member of the medical establishment qualified to hold an opinion on the subject.

Until 2011, many in the medical establishment believed that non-celiac gluten sensitivity was as chimerical as candidiasis. But then Alessio Fasano, head of the Center for Celiac Research at the University of Maryland, observed a significant immune response to gluten ingestion in subjects with suspected gluten sensitivity. This was the first hard evidence that the condition actually did exist. Two years later, however, Peter Gibson of Monash University in Australia found that only 8 percent of self-diagnosed gluten-sensitive individuals experienced a worsening of symptoms when gluten was added to their diet independently of another cause of similar symptoms: fermentable, poorly absorbed, short-chain carbohydrates (or FODMAPs), which are present in a wide range of foods, including apples, artichokes, and chickpeas. So while gluten sensitivity is no figment, it's also fairly rare.

The proposed linkage between celiac disease, gluten sensitivity, and other (sometimes disparate) disorders has also received some scientific validation. For example, in 2009 scientists at Cornell University observed specific antibodies to gluten in a subset of patients with schizophrenia. On the other hand, a carefully controlled 2010 study conducted by researchers at the University of Rochester found that a gluten-free diet had no effect on the symptoms of autistic children, pouring cold water on a pet theory of some parents of such children.

By this time, many experts regarded gluten hysteria as a greater problem than celiac disease and gluten sensitivity. In a review paper published in 2012, Italian researchers pleaded with their colleagues "to prevent a gluten preoccupation from evolving into the conviction that gluten is toxic for most of the population." Some scientists took this message outside the walls of the academy to the general public. In an interview for WebMD, Stefano Guandalini of the University of Chicago's Celiac Disease Center cautioned, "Someone who needs to be on a gluten-free diet and is closely monitored can benefit tremendously from it. But for everyone else this diet makes no sense."

Such efforts did little in the short term to check the spread of gluten scapegoating. A rash of articles with titles such as "Should You Go Gluten-Free?" and "Should We All Go Gluten-Free?" appeared on mainstream media websites like abcnews.com and in major newspapers including *The New York Times*. While none of these articles answered the questions they posed with a blanket affirmation, their very existence stoked the furnace of gluten scapegoating nevertheless.

The trend gained further momentum by forging alliances with other diet cults. The influential Paleo Diet creator Loren Cordain took to calling gluten an "antinutrient" and other nutrition advice givers followed suit. An antinutrient is a compound that inhibits the absorption of nutrients. It sounds like a terrible thing, but many natural foods contain antinutrients, and some antinutrients, including fiber, carry known health benefits. In any case, gluten is not an inherent antinutrient—it only becomes one in celiac sufferers. For everyone else, gluten is a plain old nutrient that the body absorbs fairly well and uses for vital functions.

In 2012, the gluten-free diet took the final step in its ascent toward the highest stratum of modern diet cults, becoming a celebrity weight-loss diet craze. In the spring of that year, pop singer Miley Cyrus credited a gluten-free diet for a conspicuous recent slimming that the paparazzi had made much of. She broke the news on her Twitter account, which had 5.4 million followers. "For everyone calling me anorexic I have a gluten and lactose allergy," she wrote. "It's not about weight it's about health. Gluten is crapppp anyway!" Years from now, this incident may be looked back on as the moment when gluten hysteria jumped the shark. But its short-term effect was to intensify the panic even more. In a follow-up tweet, Cyrus encouraged her followers to try the diet. Undoubtedly many of them did. Probably a larger number did not, yet passively accepted the notion that gluten is indeed "crapppp."

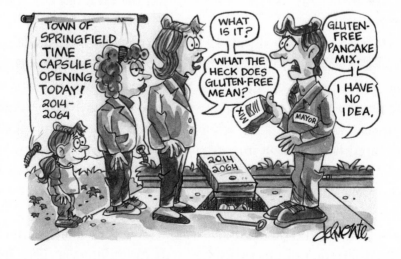

The Stress Factor

My mother stayed on the candida diet for about two and a half years. Toward the end of that term, she cheated with increasing frequency. She did so not because her willpower flagged, but rather because the diet didn't work. Her gastrointestinal symptoms simply never improved.

By the time she quit the candida diet, Laurie had begun to suspect that stress was the true cause of her suffering. She was the mother of three adolescent boys. If that wasn't stressful enough, Laurie was also working full-time as the director of the local chapter of Head Start, a gig that required her to spend fifty hours a week wrestling with grant proposals and rescuing impoverished single mothers from abusive drunken deadbeat boyfriends.

One afternoon, Laurie looked up from a grant proposal to check the time on the clock that hung from a wall of her office. A lightning bolt of panic struck her. She leapt up, gathered her things, raced out to the parking lot, and drove twenty miles to the high school my brothers and I attended. She waited and waited. No one came out. Suddenly Laurie realized that she no longer remembered which of her three boys she was supposed to pick up or if she had the time right or even the location. She burst into tears.

Soon after this incident, Laurie quit her job at Head Start. Something had to give. She began to do some things just for herself, a rarity in her life to that point. Never a lover of exercise, she took aerobics classes and even became a certified aerobics instructor. She took a few adult education courses, one of which inspired her to enroll in a graduate program in marriage and family therapy at the University of New Hampshire. By the time she received her master's degree, her gastrointestinal problems were a thing of the past.

The mind and the body are deeply interconnected. The mind is nothing more than the brain's experience of itself, after all, and the brain is a three-pound electrified hunk of flesh—part of the body. There is no separation. Because the mind is embodied, things that affect the mind affect all parts of the body. Generally speaking, factors that increase happiness enhance physical health, and factors that diminish happiness cause sickness. When we think about factors that influence health, we usually think about physical things such as diet and exercise. But mental things such as emotions and states of mind affect our overall health just as strongly.

Take anger, for example. Decades ago, researchers at Johns Hopkins Medical School asked more than a thousand of their own students to complete questionnaires designed to assess their propensity toward anger. The health of these men and women was tracked for the next thirty-six years. The angriest among them were found to be six times more likely to suffer a heart attack before age fifty-five than were the mellowest.

Social connections also have powerful effects on health. A number of studies have demonstrated that individuals with strong social relationships are healthier than more isolated persons. In one such study, more than 6,500 older adults completed surveys that were used to measure the health of their social lives. Over the next seven years, subjects classified as isolated were 26 percent more likely to die than were the most socially connected men and women.

Chronic stress—the problem my mother diagnosed in herself—is also highly damaging to physical health. The stress response is a hormonally regulated process by which the body reacts to threats. Adrenaline, cortisol, and other hormones go to work to increase heart rate, unleash energy supplies, dull pain perception, and precipitate other changes that prepare the body to make a stand or get the hell out of Dodge. This mechanism has been crucial to human survival—without it, our ancestors would have all been eaten by lions. But the stress response is tough on the body. Occasional stress episodes are easy to bounce back from, but when stressors come fast and thick and never let up, the body pays a price.

Many, but not all, of the ravages of chronic stress are linked to elevated cortisol levels. Too much cortisol exposure kills brain cells by the millions—enough to measurably reduce the overall size of the brain. It interferes with memory formation and increases the permeability of the blood-brain barrier, making the brain vulnerable to toxins it would normally be protected from. Chronic stress is believed to contribute to the development of Alzheimer's disease as well, causing indissoluble protein plaques to form in the brain. Causal relationships between stress and weight gain, heart disease, depression, and, of course, digestive disorders are well established also. It is interesting to note that irritable bowel syndrome responds especially well to placebo treatment, an indication that its origins are frequently primarily emotional.

And then we have the autoimmune diseases, of which celiac disease is but one among at least seventy. All autoimmune diseases are inflammatory in nature. Cortisol is an anti-inflammatory hormone, but chronic stress creates cortisol resistance in body tissues and thereby promotes systemic inflammation. In 2007, psychologists at King's College London established a link between childhood trauma and inflammation markers in adulthood. They concluded that more than one in ten cases of low-grade systemic inflammation in adults may be attributable to childhood trauma.

Four years later, Shanta Dube and colleagues at the Centers for Disease Control went a step further. They gathered information about "adverse childhood experiences" from more than 15,000 adults. The categories of adverse childhood experiences were physical, emotional, or sexual abuse; witnessing domestic violence; and growing up with household substance abuse, mental illness, parental divorce, and/or an incarcerated household member.

These data were used to create cumulative childhood stress scores for each subject. Dube and her colleagues then collected information from the subjects on hospitalizations for twenty-one selected autoimmune diseases in three categories. When the researchers crunched the numbers, they discovered that subjects who had suffered two or more adverse childhood experiences were between 70 and 100 percent more likely to have developed an autoimmune disease than were subjects who had suffered no adverse childhood experiences.

The incidence of all autoimmune diseases, not just celiac, has increased sharply in recent decades. So too has the amount of stress that the average person experiences in everyday life. Coincidence? Not likely. We are seeing more and more evidence that humans are not psychologically equipped to handle the world we're creating, and it's making us sick. For example, brain-imaging studies have shown that individuals who grow up in urban environments exhibit greater activity in brain regions involved in responding to threats and stress. Similar differences are seen in the brains of schizophrenics. And it so happens that people who grow up in cities are three times more likely to develop schizophrenia than are people raised in the country.

With each passing year the world becomes a little more urbanized, and as a result people become a little more stressed out and a little more likely to develop schizophrenia or another stress-related disease. The urbanization of the world is just one of many ways in which modern life is increasingly testing our psychological limits and damaging our health. Others include the disappearance of community and the deepening of social isolation, which were eloquently lamented by Robert Putnam in his book *Bowling Alone* in 2001 and have only worsened since then.

Autoimmune diseases are not genetically determined—only genetically influenced. If you have the genes for celiac disease, you may or may not actually acquire it, regardless of how much gluten you eat. Some sort of trigger is required to activate the disease. Scientists know little about these triggers, but stress is almost certainly one of them, and it could well be the big one, responsible alone for the sharply increasing rates of all autoimmune diseases as well as non-autoimmune diseases such as autism and depression and non-disease conditions, including gluten sensitivity, that are also spreading quickly.

Some experts have attributed the recent spread of celiac disease and gluten sensitivity to genetic modifications to wheat that have increased its gluten content. But this doesn't explain why autoimmune diseases generally (not to mention other diseases and conditions) are becoming more common.

What's more, wheat consumption is significantly lower than it used to be. As I noted in a previous chapter, the word "bread" is not used as a synonym for "food" in the Bible without reason. Many ancient peoples virtually did "live by bread alone." We don't know how common celiac disease was in biblical times, but we do know that as recently as the late 1960s the average American got 25 to 30 percent of his daily calories from bread. So even if there was less gluten in wheat back then, people were ingesting more gluten than they are now. It was only after bread consumption and gluten intake started to fall off that celiac disease and gluten sensitivity became more widespread.

In short, gluten is not the problem. Whatever is making people have trouble digesting gluten is the problem. In celiac patients, a genetic predisposition is a latent or potential issue, but even this is not a problem in itself. The triggers are the true villains, inasmuch as they make us less healthy whether or not they make it hard to digest gluten. Rising stress levels may or may not be the major trigger, but I suspect they are. The strains of life that tore up my mother's stomach and brought her to tears in the mid-1980s seem to me emblematic of what is most unhealthy about our world today.

The Blame-It-On-Diet Myth

The healthy-diet cults encourage people to see all disease as the consequence of nutritional error. The truth is that in the modern world, poor eating habits are easier to escape from than are certain features of our social environment whose effects on health are just as bad, and which in some cases may underlie our supposedly food-related health problems.

In addition to distracting us from other health problems, the diet-cult tendency to blame everything on bad diet promotes nutrient scapegoating, which in turn leads to the unnecessary avoidance of healthy foods. Like yeast before it, gluten was not the first nutrient scapegoat, and it probably won't be the last.

13

The Protein Club

I f you were born before 1985 then you probably remember the body-transformation contest craze of the early 2000s. There were dozens of them, and they were all pretty much the same: each competition was sponsored by a supplement company, lasted twelve weeks, and was judged on the basis of before-and-after photos. The first and biggest of these contests, started in 1996, was the Body-for-Life Challenge, which at its peak drew tens of thousands of entrants and awarded a grand prize of one million dollars. Among BLF's dozens of imitators was the Hot-Rox Inferno Challenge. In the spring of 2003, this twelve-week (of course) body-transformation contest drew 120 entrants and offered a grand prize of 1,000 dollars and a cool leather jacket. Sponsored by supplement maker Biotest and hosted by T-Mag (now T-Nation), an online social hub for bodybuilding enthusiasts, the Inferno Challenge attracted mostly men in their twenties, including John "Roman" Romaniello, then a nursing student at SUNY-Binghamton.

Roman's alarm clock woke him before dawn on Day One of the Challenge. He opened his eyes to find himself sprawled atop the worn mattress he had slept on throughout his child-hood in Glen Grove, Long Island, New York, but on which he slept only seasonally now that he was a college student. He threw back the covers with the same frisson of anticipation with which he'd scrambled out of the same bed on many a Christmas morning.

While his mother slumbered on in her own bedroom, Roman dressed in workout clothes he had laid out the previous evening, inserted his sparkplug body (five-foot-seven, 198 pounds) into his trusty '96 Honda Civic, and drove two miles to the Glen Cove Health and Fitness Center, arriving at six o'clock sharp.

The gym's owner was Alvin Baptista, whom Roman had known for a couple of years. Roman had been working at a summer job selling khakis at a local Gap store not long after his life-changing discovery of the bodybuilding lifestyle when a woman walked in and ordered thirty-six white polo shirts. He couldn't resist asking what they were for and was told that they would be worn by the staff of a new gym that was opening in Glen Cove. Roman wrangled an interview with the owner and was soon wearing one of those white polo shirts. Alvin had since become Roman's mentor as well as his summer boss.

Entering the gym with his own key, Roman stashed his duffel bag in a locker and picked out a treadmill for the first of three workouts he would do that day. It was to be a high-inten-sity interval training session, or HIIT, as this type of workout was universally known in the bodybuilding community. After a warm-up jog, Roman performed a series of sprints of ten to twenty seconds apiece separated by jogging recoveries of twenty to thirty seconds. It was a ball-buster, but over with quickly. Twenty minutes after he'd stepped onto the treadmill, Roman hopped off, dripping sweat, ready to hit the shower.

The Glen Cove Health and Fitness Center happened to share a wall with a small deli. Freshly soaped and shampooed, Roman slunk out the gym's back door and in the deli's. He ordered three egg whites and one half-cup of oatmeal, to which he added a scoop of chocolate protein powder. To round out the meal, he swallowed a handful of pills. One of them was Tribex, a purported testosterone-boosting supplement also made by Biotest. Its active ingredient was the herb tribulus terrestris.

Although the whole point of this contest, from its sponsor's perspective, was to create a buzz around its new Hot-Rox product, Roman had decided to delay using it until the final weeks. He had recently come off a major bulking phase and was a bit flabby—by his standards—at 12 percent body fat. His goal for the contest was to get leaner than he had ever been: 5 percent body fat. His strategy for winning the contest was to start using Hot-Rox—an ostensible fat-burner containing esoteric proprietary ingredients with names like Scalremax—when he was halfway to his goal in order to give the judges reason to conclude it was the supplement that took him the rest of the way.

In truth, Roman was not really counting on the stuff to work. Since entering the contest a few days earlier, he had spent hours planning his diet and training regimen in careful detail. Every workout was scheduled down to the last repetition. Three mornings per week he would do HIIT sessions like the one he had just completed. On the other mornings he would skip rope for twenty or thirty minutes. On Monday afternoons—starting today—he would do a weightlifting workout for the legs, emphasizing the quads. On Wednesday afternoons he would work his chest and biceps. Fridays he would go back to the legs, with an emphasis on the hamstrings and glutes. And on Saturdays he would hit his back and shoulders. Each night he would perform twenty-five to forty minutes of moderate-intensity cardio. All told, he'd work out twelve hours a week.

The hard piece would be the diet. In the first part of the contest, Roman would maintain a daily energy deficit of 500 calories. He knew that the closer he got to his goal, the harder it would be to lose any more fat, so in the last part of the contest he would increase his energy deficit to between 800 and 1,000 calories per day, which is equal to the deficits that physicians once prescribed to morbidly obese patients (in the days before Lap-Band surgery) when their weight was judged an immediate medical emergency.

Roman's macronutrient intake was dialed in to the gram. He would consume 100 grams of carbohydrate per day, or about a third of the amount that the average American male takes in. All of those carbs would come immediately after workouts, mostly in supplements, to refuel his depleted muscles. In the bodybuilding world, carbs were good for this and nothing more. Fat, another barely necessary evil, would be restricted to about fifty grams, and almost all of it would come from flaxseed oil. The remaining 1,200 calories of Roman's initial 2,000-calorie daily allotment would come from protein. According to the World Health Organization, a person must get at least 10 percent of his or her calories from protein to be healthy. The typical American diet is 18 percent protein. In clinical research, a 30-percent protein diet is classified as high-protein. John Romaniello's contest diet was 60 percent protein.

Make a Muscle

Athletes have used high-protein diets to fortify their muscles for centuries. Of course, nobody thought of these diets explicitly as high-protein before proteins were actually discovered in the nineteenth century. Instead, athletes before the turn of the last century attributed the muscle-building effects of high-protein foods to other qualities. Meat was regarded as a good muscle builder because meat itself was muscle. According to one ancient account, in 480 B.C.E. the Greek runner Dromeus of Stymphalos won a pair of Olympic footraces after eating nothing but meat for ten months. Afterward, his diet was widely emulated by other athletes. One of the most legendary sportsmen of ancient times was the Italian wrestler Milo of Croton, who won six times in seven Olympiads and was said to eat twenty pounds of meat every day.

A Swedish chemist named Jöns Jakob Berzelius discovered protein in 1838, adapting the Greek word proteios (meaning "first importance") to name it. Initially protein was wrongly credited as the primary source of energy for muscle work. Among the most notable proponents of this theory was the German chemist Justus von Liebig, who in 1840 developed a high-protein meat extract that he later commercialized as a nutritional supplement. While not marketed to athletes specifically, Liebig's Meat Extract became popular among them.

A couple of Liebig's English contemporaries proved that protein in fact contributes far less energy to exercise than do both fat and carbohydrate, but force of habit ensured that high-protein diets remained prevalent in sports nevertheless. In the 1940s, these diets got a new justification. A series of studies conducted by German researchers demonstrated that weightlifters gained more muscle mass and strength when they consumed more protein. It made sense: muscle tissue is roughly 25 percent protein. (Most of the rest is water.) Therefore, muscles grow primarily by incorporating more protein into their structure. Weightlifting creates a biochemical demand for new muscle tissue. Dietary protein supplies the raw materials to satisfy this demand.

At about the same time these discoveries were made, the body-building subculture was born. Charles Atlas is recognized as the man who fathered the modern male mania for getting huge. His iconic advertisements for a booklet that detailed the exercise and dietary methods that transformed him from a "98-pound weak-ling" into "the world's most perfectly developed man" became ubiquitous in comic books of the 1940s. His dietary secrets to muscle-building were immortalized in "The Charles Atlas Song" of *The Rocky Horror Picture Show*: "He'll eat nutritious high protein and swallow raw eggs."

By the time Arnold Schwarzenegger brought bodybuilding into the American mainstream in the 1970s, protein had become an obsession among seekers of hugeness. Schwarzenegger ate up to 350 grams (or 1,400 calories) of protein a day during his reign as Mr. Universe. It's not easy to get that much protein from regular food. You'd have to eat sixty eggs a day to get Arnie's requisite 350 grams.

Or you could drink a protein shake—an alternative that became viable in the early 1990s, when food chemists figured out how to cheaply extract nearly pure whey protein from cow's milk. The first person to capitalize on this opportunity was David Jenkins, a British expatriate and former Olympic sprinter who had just been released from federal prison after serving a short sentence for masterminding a hundred-million-dollar steroid-trafficking operation. Seeing a chance to go legit, Jenkins founded a company called Next Proteins just north of San Diego. Its flagship product, Designer Whey, a flavored powdered protein drink mix, made Jenkins a millionaire all over again and helped create a multibillion-dollar bodybuilding-supplements industry. Designer Whey contains more than four times as much protein per serving as an egg.

Thanks in large measure to the marketing of such products, the belief that very high levels of protein intake are needed to maximize muscle growth has become an article of faith in body-building and strength-based sports. In 2011, researchers at St. Louis University surveyed forty-two strength-trained male college athletes about their perceptions of protein requirements. These athletes estimated their protein requirement to be about 2.4 grams per kilogram of body weight daily, or double the amount of protein that the average American adult consumes. One third of those surveyed believed that a supplement was required to meet their protein needs.

They were wrong on all counts. The latest science has stuck a pin in the idea that athletes need to pound protein to get huge. While there is an advantage to eating more than the recommended daily intake of 0.8 grams per kilogram of body weight daily, there is no benefit to eating in excess of the 1.2 grams per kilogram that the typical American diet provides. In 1992, Mark Tarnopolsky and colleagues at McMaster University administered diets that provided a daily allotment of either 1.35 or 2.62 grams of protein per kilogram of body weight to previously untrained men who were subjected to one month of intensive weightlifting (ninety minutes a day, six days a week). Both groups gained muscle size and strength, but those who consumed the larger amount of protein gained no more than those who took in scarcely half as much.

What's more, research suggests that experienced bodybuilders who have already gotten huge actually need *less* protein to maintain their existing muscle mass than beginning weightlifters need to beef up in the first place. That's because weightlifting teaches the body to retain more protein from the diet. Ironically, massive protein intake partially counteracts this adaptation, increasing protein turnover and thus creating a kind of dependency on continued massive protein intake. A protein-gobbling bodybuilder deprived of his protein shakes might indeed start to lose muscle even though he never needed the shakes to get huge to begin with.

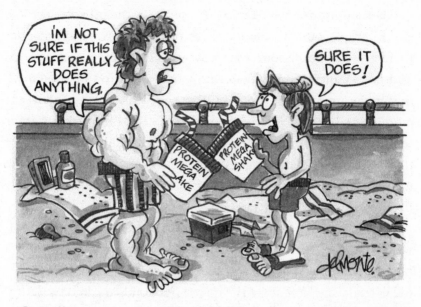

One dietary practice of bodybuilders that actually has been validated by science is the ritual of taking in a dose of protein soon after a workout, as most bodybuilders do with their shakes. The muscles are able to use dietary protein to build new muscle tissue more effectively at this time than at any other time. But the maximum amount of protein that the body can possibly make use of within this window is ten grams, or less than half the amount of protein in a typical shake and about the same amount of protein in a plain old turkey sandwich.

Despite their meathead reputation, many bodybuilders are well read in the scientific literature, and they have seen the studies that threaten to invalidate the protein doctrine. To preserve this doctrine they have put forward a number of counterarguments. One of them is the "insurance" argument. According to this line of reasoning, while consuming a ton of protein may be no better than eating a normal amount of protein, it's also no worse. And since everyone agrees that a normal amount of protein is better than a little, a guy might as well consume a ton of protein just to be extra sure he's getting enough to maximize muscle development.

Another argument that is used to preserve the protein doctrine is the "displacement" theory. This one reminds naysayers that there are only three sources of energy in the diet: protein, carbs, and fat. While bodybuilders may not need a ton of protein to maximize muscle development, they certainly don't need to eat a ton of carbs or fat. Bodybuilders are better off satisfying their total energy requirement by eating more protein than necessary than they are by eating more carbs or fat than necessary because, calorie for calorie, protein is more filling and is therefore less likely to be converted to body fat.

The more stereotypical meathead tends to favor the "real-world" argument. This argument points out that all of the hugest bodybuilders eat tons of protein. Who cares what the pipsqueaks in lab coats say? Whatever the hugest bodybuilders do is by definition what works best. One senses that this is the counterargument that all bodybuilders believe most fervently in their hearts.

Secret Identity

John Romaniello spent fifteen hours of Day One of the 2003 Hot-Rox Inferno Challenge at the Glen Cove Health and Fitness Club. This was not unusual. He spent almost every waking moment of every day there. After all, he worked at the club. When he wasn't working out himself, he was either training clients or manning the front desk. Most of his friends were members too, so Roman could satisfy his need for social interaction under the same roof. There was no other place he really cared to be.

Growing up, Roman had never seemed destined to become a gym rat. Short and chubby, he filled his free time with video-games and Dungeons & Dragons, taking up sports only when a guidance counselor suggested that diversifying his resume would help Roman—a straight-A student—get into a good college. So he wrestled and played football and ran track and got into Cornell. (He would later transfer to Binghamton.)

During his freshman year in Ithaca, Roman glanced at a recent photograph of himself and reeled in horror. The pudgy little wuss he saw was not the person he saw himself as. A switch was flipped inside him. Roman decided to get in shape—*great* shape. Nerd that he was, he did not immediately go for a run or swear off meat for a month. Instead, he studied. Roman read every book and every magazine on weightlifting and muscle-building nutrition he could get his hands on. He started with mainstream stuff like *Arnold Schwarzenegger's Encyclopedia of Bodybuilding* and *Men's Fitness* magazine, then went online and discovered hardcore gurus like Arthur Jones, Mike Mentzer, and Ellington Darden. He developed a plan that synthesized the teachings that most appealed to him, and within a few months he no longer looked anything like the pudgy little wuss in that photograph. It was a Charles Atlas story writ for the twenty-first century.

Roman's new lifestyle took him happily out of step with those around him. No one else he knew ate six meals a day or worked out twice a day. Roman imagined himself as a kind of interloper, like a spy behind enemy lines or an alien in human disguise. He alone now possessed a carnal wisdom which he vaguely pitied others for lacking. But while he enjoyed the gentle superiority of the saved among the lost, he was also a bit lonely—until he met Alvin Baptista.

Through his new mentor, Roman learned that a robust body-building subculture existed, and was initiated into it. The older man taught the younger the lingo, the customs, and the attitude. It was Alvin also who directed Roman to T-Mag, where his personal awakening was fully consummated. Among the first articles Roman chanced upon there was one written by T-Mag editor T. C. Luoma and titled "The Secret Culture." Luoma wrote about how bodybuilders were like superheroes with secret identities—doctors and salesmen and carpenters by day who tore off their disguises in the gym at night to reveal their secret selves. Roman thirstily imbibed the message. He realized suddenly that there were thousands of other men like him, men who felt like misunderstood freaks in society, who suffered impatiently through school and work as though life as everyone else knew it were nothing but a distraction from true life, the life of bench presses and protein shakes and muscle magazines.

T-Mag became a new outlet for the expression of Roman's secret self. He spent hours on its thriving forums, boasting about his latest numbers, requesting advice, and making friends. Many of these friendships migrated offline, affording Roman the satisfaction of regular face-to-face interaction with fellow members of the Secret Culture. Within a couple of years, Roman himself was writing for T-Mag and giving advice to the next generation of newbies. He resolved to turn his hobby into a profession. His ambitions were large: to become a world-class personal trainer, a famous workout guru, and an envied fitness model. (Roman's mug had always photographed well, even when he was chubby.) When T. C. Luoma personally invited Roman to participate in the Hot-Rox Inferno Challenge, the young dreamer accepted the offer wholeheartedly, seeing in it an opportunity to move a step closer to his destiny. All he had to do was win.

The weightlifting and cardio workouts Roman did in the challenge, the high-protein meals he ate, and the supplements he took were more than just tools that he believed in to secure his destiny. They were more than a synthesis of the best methods Roman had learned in his two years of total intellectual and physical immersion in bodybuilding. They were also rituals of belonging to the Secret Culture that now supplied a big chunk of Roman's identity. Doing the workouts and eating the meals and supplements—and looking the way these things made him look—identified Roman as "one of us" in the eyes of other Secret Culture members and gave Roman a reassuring sense of having found his place in the world.

At midmorning on Day One of the Inferno Challenge, Roman consumed his second meal. "Meal" is probably not the best word to describe the repast, because it consisted of a protein shake. At noon, Roman ate the lunch he would eat almost every day throughout the challenge: three grilled chicken breasts and a side of steamed vegetables. It was either that or tuna straight from the can.

In the late afternoon, after training his last client of the day, Roman hit the weights. He did five sets of barbell squats and a few other leg exercises, using so much weight that other gym-goers couldn't help but pause their own workouts to sneak sidelong looks at him. When his quads were good and fried, Roman did a three-part cardio workout involving stair climbing, rowing, and skipping rope. His reward was a recovery drink—another Biotest supplement—called Low-Carb Grow.

Dinner was a bowl of cottage cheese mixed with peanut butter and chocolate protein powder. Before he went to bed, Roman took one more round of supplements, including a product called M, a supposed estrogen blocker containing ingredients such as trihydroxystilbene, tocotrienols, and Vitex agnus-castus.

He was off to a great start.

Powders, Potions, and Pills

The world's largest sports-supplement retailer is General Nutrition Centers, which operates more than 7,000 stores and whose annual sales exceed two billion dollars. A neophyte bodybuilder who walks into his local neighborhood GNC in search of products that will help him attain his goals runs the risk of being paralyzed by the paradox of choice. There are six or seven different kinds of creatine to build muscles, an equal number of amino acid supplements, arginine-based nitric oxide boosters that are purported to create a "pumped look," testosterone boosters including DHEA and HMB, aids to anaerobic metabolism such as beta-alanine, pre-workout stimulants with names like Jacked and Force Factor, so-called "thermogenics" for fat-burning, and more.

Exactly one of these supplements really works: creatine. Because it works, roughly half of all males who lift weights, whether for sports or as recreational bodybuilders, take or have taken creatine supplements. Creatine is a compound that is manufactured in the body and stored in the muscles to provide energy for very high-intensity muscle work. Small amounts of creatine are also obtained through the diet from meat. Twenty-five years ago, virtually no one outside the ivory tower had ever heard of creatine, but scientists knew that it played a role in high-intensity muscle work. Then, in 1992, a team of Swedish researchers published a study reporting that creatine supplementation greatly increased muscle creatine stores in subjects who engaged in resistance exercise.

This study caused little fanfare because it did not look at any possible benefit of creatine supplementation. But a savvy nutritional biochemist in California named Anthony Alameda latched onto it, formed a company called EAS (which stood for Experimental and Applied Sciences), and began to market creatine supplements to bodybuilders. He was prescient. Within a year, new research had shown that creatine supplementation significantly increased the muscles' capacity for high-intensity work.

Alameda was also a sharp businessman. He approached Bill Phillips, the young publisher of a Colorado-based meathead magazine called *Muscle Media*, and invited him to become a partner in the business. A former steroid user who had authored the definitive underground manual on steroid use, Phillips tried creatine, realized that it actually worked, and quickly jumped on board. The first creatine supplement, called Phosphagen, soon hit the market. Early customers were shocked to discover that they did not have to talk themselves into believing this new stuff was really doing something. Word spread and the new business partners quickly amassed a fortune.

Phillips made a second fortune when he wrote *Body-for-Life*, a book that served as a promotional vehicle for the physique transformation contest of the same name, which was organized by EAS and served to promote its supplements. The title sold more than four million copies in its first four years in print, becoming the best-selling fitness book in history.

The runaway success of creatine supplementation attracted the attention of exercise and nutrition scientists, who in the decade after its advent cumulatively subjected creatine to greater scientific scrutiny than any other supplement had ever been subjected to. It passed every test. Creatine's ability to magnify the gains in muscle strength and mass that resulted from resistance training were reconfirmed. The compound was also found to increase performance in repeated bouts of high-intensity work such as multiple sprints. Even nonathletes may benefit from creatine supplementation, which has been shown to attenuate muscle loss associated with muscle-wasting diseases, bed rest, and aging. The safety of creatine supplementation has been thoroughly defended. Its only side effect is water retention.

Another predictable effect of creatine's success was a feverish search among sports-supplement makers for "the next creatine." Many candidates have been put forward, but none so far has survived rigorous examination. The same process is repeated over and over: First some esoteric compound gets promising results in a single study. Then one or more companies (usually more, given the intensity of competition in today's sports-supplement industry) scramble to bring supplemental forms of that compound to market. As these supplements are being sold and used, their active ingredient is subjected to additional scientific scrutiny. Almost always, these tests fail to substantiate the promise shown in the original study. Science concludes that the supplement is essentially useless. The manufacturers respond to this bad news by continuing to make and sell their products, highlighting the few studies yielding positive results in their marketing and ignoring the much larger number of studies yielding negative results. Bodybuilders and athletes continue to buy the products.

Often the scientist who discovers the muscle-building effects of some esoteric compound and the businessman who profits from bringing it to market as a dietary supplement are the same person. One of the earliest supplements to be touted as "the next creatine" was beta-hydroxy beta-methylbutyrate. HMB was discovered in the mid-1990s by Steve Nissen, a researcher at Iowa State University who also headed a company called Metabolic Technologies. In 1996, Nissen authored a study reporting that HMB supplementation had been found to significantly increase the benefits of weightlifting compared to placebo. Metabolic Technologies took out six patents on HMB and licensed the right to manufacture it and to cite Nissen's research to several sports supplement brands.

Other researchers were critical of the design of Nissen's first and subsequent studies on HMB. They conducted their own tests and, more often than not, obtained negative results. In 2009, scientists in New Zealand published a comprehensive review of the research on HMB. They concluded that HMB accelerates strength gains in beginners who have just peeled themselves off the couch to start a weightlifting program, but is completely useless for those who have been at it for a while. In other words, HMB will make you stronger somewhat faster, but ultimately it will make you no stronger than you could become without it. Yet HMB remains a fairly popular supplement among the hardcore gym rats it benefits least.

Join the Club

Midway through the 2003 Hot-Rox Inferno Challenge, John Romaniello suffered a setback. He was preparing to do a set of dumbbell chest presses with a pair of 100-pound weights. When he attempted to lift the dumbbells off the floor, a searing bolt of pain shot through his left wrist. Roman had become so strong that his joints now had trouble handling some of the loads that his freakishly powerful muscles moved with ease. He had severely sprained his wrist and would be unable to use it to do much of anything for three weeks.

Roman modified his training as best he could to work around the problem. He replaced his dumbbell chest presses with seated machine flyes, where loading occurred at the elbow instead of at the wrist. He replaced the lat pull-downs that he normally did to build his back muscles with machine lat pullovers where loading again occurred at the elbow.

On May 31, the last day of the challenge, Roman had a complete battery of measurements taken as well as a series of "after" photos. Despite the setback, his program had been a smashing success. He lost thirteen pounds of body fat, gained four pounds of muscle, and lowered his body fat percentage from 12.0 to 5.7. Roman had looked shredded already when he started the challenge, but in his "after" photos he looked like an anatomical diagram of human musculature.

Roman was on vacation in Maine when he found out he had won the contest. His companions in Kennebunk were three other young rising stars of the Secret Culture: Joel Marion, who had won the 2001 Body-for-Life contest; Eric Cressey, who at age twenty-two was already on his way toward becoming one of the nation's leading rehabilitative strength coaches for athletes; and Eric Chessen, who is recognized today as the preeminent authority on fitness for the autistic. Roman had made his way to the very center of the subculture that defined him, winning the respect of those he most respected within that world. He and his new friends were the cool kids, the popular guys, their near-perfect bodies the envy of thousands of other young men who would hang on their every word in the hope of replicating their results.

Even more valuable than the thousand-dollar check and the cool leather jacket Roman got for winning the Hot-Rox Inferno Challenge was a lengthy victory interview that he gave for T-Mag, which served as a platform for his budding career as a body-transformation guru. In that interview, Roman discussed the finer points of his training, mentioning his use of "Staley's EDT" and "Meltdown Training." Such terms would have been utterly meaningless to outsiders but were familiar to all T-Mag regulars. Roman also discussed the minutiae of his winning diet, noting his implementation of "Massive Eating," "refeeding," and "overfeeding" techniques. These terms as well were like secret handshakes of the Secret Culture, vocabulary that all body-builders either knew or pretended to know until they were able to learn it on the sly.

After winning the contest, Roman sent his "after" photos to fitness modeling agencies. He got several callbacks and eventually signed with Fusion Management. His career as a trainer took off. Upon graduating from SUNY-Binghamton, Roman moved to Manhattan to set up shop. By virtue of his knowledge, his physique, his celebrity within the Secret Culture, and his connections, Roman quickly built up a large and diverse clientele of personal-training clients. He continued to write for T-Nation and also scored bylines in *Men's Fitness*, *Shape*, and other glossy magazines. Later, he began to produce multimedia training and diet programs, including the popular Final Phase Fat Loss, which was based in part on the things he learned during the Inferno Challenge.

It's been a while since Roman subjected himself to anything quite as intense as that contest. He still trains hard, eats carefully, and looks good enough to model. But he no longer logs twelve hours of exercise every week and he eats a lot more real food than he did before. One reason is that he can afford to buy real food now; a second is that he learned how to cook. If Roman wants a high-protein dinner, he'll skip the protein shake and cook up a nice steak instead.

Only two supplements remain in Roman's pill regimen: creatine and Biotest's Alpha Male, which is basically a repackaged version of its old Tribex product. But he often forgets to take the latter, while he never forgets to take his creatine.

The Because-It-Works Myth

Every meal is a ritual of sorts. No matter what we eat or how we eat it, we've probably done it a thousand times before—and if we haven't, others surely have. All habits, including meals, become part of who we are. They also bind us together with others who practice the same rituals. Some meals are more ritualistic than others. A Passover Seder, for example, is a meal that makes a Jew highly conscious of his Jewishness, whereas the pickled herring he may eat once or twice a week does not, though it too connects him to his heritage.

Healthy-diet cults make each meal more explicitly ritualistic than it would otherwise be for the average member of our society. When a bodybuilder drinks a protein shake or swallows muscle-building pills or eats tuna straight out of the can, he is conscious of his identity as a bodybuilder and as a member of the Secret Culture. The ritual of juicing does the same for the raw-foodist and that of counting points does the same for the Weight Watchers dieter.

If you ask a longtime member of any healthy-diet cult why he eats the way he does, he will probably say something to the effect of "Because it works." This is true as far as it goes. Seasoned followers of diet cults are almost invariably satisfied with the results they're getting. But what they're often deceived about is the fact that the particular diet they follow is not necessary to the attainment of those results. Bodybuilders could pack on just as much muscle on a diet that did not require protein-gobbling or supplement-guzzling. Followers of other diet cults also could get results comparable to those they're currently enjoying from somewhat different ways of eating.

There's an irony here. Diet-cult members believe they are eating more pragmatically than the rest of us do, when in fact they are eating more ritualistically. They see the protein shake as a necessary means to the desired end of building muscle, when in fact it is a sacrament.

14

What's Your Poison?

Most philosophers do not write about their diet. That's because most philosophers do not believe that what they eat is relevant to their philosophy. But Friedrich Nietzsche was not most philosophers.

Nietzsche's penultimate book, written in 1888, was a strange career retrospective that in some ways foreshadowed his plunge into syphilitic madness a year later. The second chapter, titled "Why I Am So Clever," contained a lengthy disquisition on the author's dietary preferences. Nietzsche informed his readers that he grew up eating "very badly" and that he was amazed at how long it took him to attain his "maximum of strength" in body and mind with food choices that really worked for him.

Although he was born and raised in Germany, Nietzsche scorned the German diet, calling it the world's worst, even more pitiful than the English diet.

"The best cuisine is that of Piedmont," he opined, referring to Italy's mountainous northwest region, famous for its truffles, dried meats, cheeses, and egg-rich pastas. (Nietzsche was residing in Turin, Piedmont's largest city, when he wrote these words.)

Hearty meals were easier to digest than small ones, Nietzsche believed, and snacking between meals was best avoided. "One must," he wrote, "know the size of one's stomach."

When he was approaching middle age, Nietzsche briefly experimented with vegetarianism. The diet produced no palpable benefits and so, he said, he was easily persuaded to return to meat-eating by his composer friend Richard Wagner, whose music sounds to me like the music of a meat lover.

Alcohol did not agree with Nietzsche. Even a single glass of wine or beer turned his life into a "vale of misery." He drank only pure water (carrying a canteen everywhere he went) and a little strong tea in the morning. Coffee, he stated, "spreads darkness."

Having exhausted the topic of his eating habits, Nietzsche moved on to other elements of his lifestyle, describing in minute detail his preferences in the matters of habitation, weather, and physical exercise. (Nietzsche was a strong swimmer and a prodigious walker.) Anticipating the reader's obvious question—"Why the heck is this self-styled 'antichrist' (for so he was) introducing a review of his life and work by boring us with a litany of the finer points of his way of life?"—he preemptively answered it.

"These small things," he wrote—"nutrition, place, climate, exercise, the whole casuistry of selfishness—are inconceivably more important than everything one has taken to be important so far."

Nietzsche was talking about health. Health, he believed, was more important than anything else one had taken to be important.

Of course, people everywhere have always been concerned about their health, but before Nietzsche embarked upon his mission to "revaluate all values," as he phrased it, other things (such as God, the common good, happiness) had always been considered more important. Nietzsche was the first thinker to proclaim that *nothing* was more important than one's own health—that health was, in fact, the purpose of life.

You don't have to look very far to find the source of this world-view. It grew straight from the soil of Nietzsche's life experience, particularly his never-ending fight with infirmities. His father, a Lutheran minister, died at the age of thirty-six of a horrific brain disease, which his son may have inherited. While still in grade school, Nietzsche began to experience migraine headaches, a condition that would plague him for the remainder of his days. A medicine he took to treat the migraines caused nausea and indigestion. During a brief military stint, Nietzsche suffered a bad riding accident that rendered him unfit for further service. When he was thirty-five, his failing health forced him to resign his position as professor of philology at the University of Basel. Nine years later, he collapsed on a street in Turin while trying to defend a stranger's horse against an unmerited flogging. Nietzsche passed the next decade in a mental asylum in a vegetative state and died when he was fifty-five.

Despite these many vicissitudes, Nietzsche found the where-withal to make something beautiful of his life, writing monu-mental books that will endure forever and filling the too-few years allotted to him with rich experiences. The success of Nietzsche's brave-faced struggle to realize his potential in the face of the Job-like sequence of misfortunes visited upon him transformed his outlook on life. "I took myself in hand," he wrote. "I made myself healthy again. I discovered life anew, including myself; I tasted all good and even little things as others cannot easily taste them—I turned my will to health, to *life*, into a philosophy."

This philosophy was shaped by more than personal overcoming. Like all philosophies, Nietzsche's was also a product of its time. Specifically, his was flavored by the influence of Charles Darwin's theory of the origin of species. Nietzsche was the first great philosopher to emerge after Darwin, with the stroke of a pen, turned humans into animals—a species of ape, to be precise. While Nietzsche's few explicit references to Darwin in his writings were caustic, the evolutionist's imprint on his thinking was obvious. A philosopher's duty is to tell people what to live for and how best to live. Nietzsche accepted the Darwinian premise that a human being was an animal like any other animal, and this led him to conclude that the purpose of human life was the same as the purpose of the life of any animal: to become as healthy as possible—"dangerously healthy," in the ideal scenario—for its own sake.

Nietzsche recognized, however, that humans were a unique sort of animal. Unlike the rest of the animal kingdom, people had ideas. Yet the realm of ideas, Nietzsche saw, was just another dimension through which humans pursued greater health. The pet ideas of each man were those he discovered to be most *nourishing* to him. A man believed what it was good for him to believe. Even the most abstract ideas that a person held in special favor were rooted in his bodily interests. There was a fundamental consistency between one's higher tastes—art, people, politics, culture—and one's dietary biases.

"All prejudices come from the intestines," Nietzsche wrote.

The optimal diet for each person therefore was the collection of specific foods and eating patterns which most enlarged his physical health *and* best expressed his overall nature. As such, this diet was unique—at least in its finer details—for each person. To become as healthy as one could be—and to become most fully oneself—a person had to discover his optimal personal diet through experience, as Nietzsche himself had done.

"For ordinary purposes it may be formulated as follows," he wrote: "How precisely must you feed yourself so as to be able to attain to the maximum of strength, of virtú in the Renaissance style—of virtue free from moralistic acid?"

This stomach-led project of personal development was one crucial part of a larger journey toward total health that Nietzsche urged everyone to undertake. Each person was born with a unique nature and potential, he believed. To fully realize this potential, the individual needed to discern the things in the world that best nourished his unique nature toward full maturity, and one did this by exploring his tastes in all things.

According to Nietzsche's holistic philosophy of individual health, we "become ourselves" by learning which foods agree with us and which do not, by discovering our useful talents, by understanding which sorts of people we like being around and which sorts we cannot abide, by knowing how we prefer to entertain and restore ourselves, and so on. Each of us has a different blueprint for complete mind–body health. What works for me won't necessarily work for you.

Diet is no exception. The dietary rules that Nietzsche shared in his next-to-last book were *his* rules. They were not rules for others, or even recommendations. The only thing Nietzsche recommended was that everyone discover his own rules. He made this point often in his work—in general reference to his values—and he made it once more near the end of his lucid life in specific reference to diet:

"Everybody has his own measure," he wrote, "often between the narrowest and most delicate limits."

Cults of Dietary Individuality

Friedrich Nietzsche's idea that each person has his own best diet proved to be remarkably prescient. More than a century after he articulated it, genetic mapping demonstrated that, lo and behold, no single way of eating is best for every person. Scientists have coined the term "nutritional genomics" to refer to the study of the genetically based individuality of human nutritional needs. The basic goal of the field is to gather enough knowledge about how genes interact with diet to enable clinicians to give patients custom dietary recommendations that will minimize certain health risks. No one in the field expects that there will come a day when doctors can tell a person exactly what and how much to eat for breakfast, lunch, and dinner every day to attain his or her personal "maximum of health." Everything we know about the human body to this point suggests that any number of different diets will yield good health for the average person. Yet most experts do expect that eventually it will be possible to tease out a few specific dietary rules that apply to some people and not others based on their genetic makeup.

For example, scientists have identified certain genetic variations that allow a person to eat a high-fat diet without getting fat, and they've found certain other genes that have the opposite effect. Should you learn that you possess the latter and not the former, presumably you would want to put yourself on a low-fat diet. If, on the other hand, you were to learn that you possess only the protective genes, you would be free to choose either a high-fat or a low-fat diet.

The scientific discovery of metabolic individuality, which confirmed Friedrich Nietzsche's nineteenth-century intuition, struck a devastating blow against the healthy-diet cults' presumption that there is one perfect diet for everyone. But it wasn't a death blow. After all, who says you can't make a diet cult out of the very idea of nutritional individuality?

A number of enterprising diet gurus have done just that. Unfortunately, the various cults of dietary individuality that have popped up in recent decades share a common flaw, which is a tendency to greatly exaggerate the individuality of human nutritional needs. The preachers of dietary individuality talk as though the various "metabolic types" of humans were as unalike as different species in terms of their nutritional needs. In reality, genetic nuances aside, all humans share the same basic nutritional requirements. Science has succeeded in defining a general dietary framework that works for everybody. Individual differences certainly do exist, but they lie at the margins, whereas the core requirements are universal.

The cults of dietary individuality also give DNA too much credit as the source of individual dietary needs. For that matter, so do some scientists. Nietzsche, on the other hand, recognized that a person's optimal individual diet was defined by his mind as much as it was by his body, and that this way of eating served to shape identity as much as it did to strengthen the vital organs.

Notable among the preachers of dietary individuality is James D'Adamo, a naturopathic doctor who developed the theory that the ideal diet for each person was determined by one's blood type. His son Peter popularized the theory with a series of books that included the mega-bestseller *Eat Right 4 Your Type*. According to the D'Adamos' theory, people with blood type A should be mostly vegetarian; those with blood type B should eat a little of everything; those with blood type AB should eat lots of seafood and dairy; and those with blood type O should eat lots of meat. The organizing principle behind these dietary prescriptions was that a person of a given blood type ought to eat in a way that borrowed key features from traditional diets that existed in parts of the world where each of the four blood types originated.

As you see, this theory is a rather tortured way of stopping one step short of suggesting that individuals who belong to a particular ethnic group ought to eat the traditional diet of their people. One could make a reasonably solid argument that the traditional diet of the ethnic group a person belongs to is a good place to start in the search for a personalized healthy diet. For example, dairy is not a traditional part of the diet for many people in Asia, and thus a lot of Asians have difficulty digesting lactose or are lactose-intolerant. But James and Peter D'Adamo wanted their theory to feel more *scientific*, so they wedged in blood types as a conceptual middleman. The irony, of course, is that this arbitrary insertion made their theory *less* scientific than the commonsense version of the hypothesis would have been, because there isn't a shred of scientific evidence of a link between blood type and individual dietary needs.

The glue that binds together nutrition, blood type, and health outcomes in the D'Adamos' theory is a class of compounds called lectins. Lectins are proteins that have a strong affinity for sugars. They are present in small amounts in a wide variety of plant and animal foods, and they serve a host of functions in the human body, almost all of which entail binding to sugar molecules. One job of lectins is to control the concentration of platelets (which influence bleeding and clotting) in the blood. Since 1945 it has been known that some lectins are blood-type-specific. James and Peter D'Adamo seized on this discovery to argue that certain lectins in foods are compatible with one or more specific blood types and are incompatible with one or more others. Stretching the science even further, they contended that consuming lectins which were not compatible with one's blood type caused all kinds of health problems, from anemia to cancer.

The *real* scientists who performed the studies on which this theory was very loosely based did not themselves endorse it. According to their own interpretation of their research, dietary lectins have the same effects—some beneficial, others potentially harmful—in *all* humans. The issue of blood-type specificity in lectins is inconsequential. What's more, the harm (such as damage to the intestinal wall) that lectins may cause happens only when lectins are consumed in tremendous excess.

The mainstream scientific position on blood type-based diets was bluntly summarized by Victor Herbert, a hematologist at Mt. Sinai

Medical Center, in a CNN interview. "It's pure horse manure," he said. "It has no relation to reality. The genes for blood type have nothing to do with the genes that handle the food we eat."

The blood-type diet enjoyed a brief period of great popularity in the late 1990s, but it has since faded into obscurity. By contrast, the original individualistic diet cult—known as metabolic typing—remains quite popular. Metabolic typing was conceived by a dentist named William Kelley in the 1960s. In 1970, Kelley was convicted of practicing medicine without a license. In spite of this blow to his credibility, Kelley's brainchild survived, and more than thirty years later his chief apostle, Bill Wolcott, wrote a book titled *The Metabolic Typing Diet* that greatly expanded his mentor's cult following.

The basic premise of Wolcott's Metabolic Typing Diet is that macronutrient needs vary drastically between individuals. The specific proportions of proteins, carbohydrates, and fats in the diet that best support the health of one person might destroy the health of another person. (The first chapter of Wolcott's book is titled "One Man's Food Is Another's Poison.") Like the father-son team of James and Peter D'Adamo, Bill Wolcott believes that individual differences in dietary needs originated in the diverse ancestral diets that sprang up around the world after the Journey of Man ended. But whereas the D'Adamos identified four categories of dietary needs based on blood types, Wolcott named three categories based on unspecified genetic variations. (The human genome had not been fully mapped when Wolcott wrote his book, so he was spared the need to specify the relevant genes.) According to Wolcott, some people thrive on lots of protein, others are healthiest when they eat plenty of carbohydrate, and the rest function best on a balanced-macronutrient diet.

If it were true that each person could be healthiest on one and only one of these three diets, the way to prove it would be to conduct a large-scale controlled study in which subjects were cycled through all three diets under supervision. If there was a clear pattern of some people getting healthier on the high-protein diet and less healthy on the high-carb and mixed diets, others getting healthier on the high-carb diet and less healthy on the high-protein and mixed diets, and still others getting healthier on the mixed diet and less healthy on the high-protein and high-carb diets, Wolcott's theory would be confirmed. No such study has ever been done. But lots of existing research offers strong evidence that such a study would blow up in Wolcott's face if it ever were conducted.

Within the past fifteen years, geneticists have identified a long list of genes that affect the metabolism of carbs, fats, and proteins. The majority of these genes exist in all humans (not to mention other primates), which means that they entered the genome and spread throughout our species before the Journey of Man even started and haven't been displaced in any ethnic subpopulation within the last 60,000 years. Therefore, the macronutrient needs of all humans are basically the same.

Epidemiological research supports this genetic evidence. For example, it has been established that a diet in which protein supplies 10 percent of total calories is sufficient to support normal health in 98 percent of the population. We also know that nearly everyone can tolerate a protein intake as high as 35 percent. So not only do all humans share the same general macronutrient needs, but those universally shared needs are far broader than the rules of the Metabolic Typing Diet.

Genetically based differences in carbohydrate, fat, and protein metabolism do exist, but these differences don't support the Metabolic Typing Diet's division of the human population into three tidy dietary buckets. I mentioned earlier that scientists have identified gene variations that protect some people against the fattening effect of high-fat diets. One of these genes is known as APOA5. In a recent study, roughly 13 percent of subjects were found to have a variation of this gene that kept them from becoming overweight when they got more than 30 percent of their energy from fat. The remaining 87 percent had variations of the gene that would cause them to pork up when their fat intake exceeded the 30 percent threshold. But everyone, whatever their APOA5 status, is healthy on a diet that is at least 20 percent fat. So the official recommended fat-intake range of 20 to 35 percent of total calories (endorsed by the Institute of Medicine) is truly one-size-fits-all.

The Metabolic Typing Diet was developed at a time when the popular-diet culture was obsessed with macronutrient ratios, so it's not surprising that it shares that focus. But if the Metabolic Typing Diet had been founded upon real knowledge of genetically based differences in individual nutritional needs, its focus would have been much broader, encompassing micronutrient needs as well. Since Wolcott's book was published in 2001, researchers have identified a number of genes that affect individual vitamin and mineral requirements. Yet even these differences do not create a need for radically different individual diets.

For example, Steven Zeisel at the University of North Carolina has demonstrated that particular genetic variations determine how much choline (a B-complex vitamin) individuals need. The recommended minimum intake of choline is 500 mg per day. But most premenopausal women need less because they have a lot of estrogen coursing through their veins, and this allows them to make their own choline. Some women, however, have a gene variation that negates this benefit. As a result, their choline needs remain at 500 mg per day, matching the needs of all men and postmenopausal women. It's not hard to get 500 mg of choline, which is available in a variety of foods—eggs, meat, seafood, greens, oats, potatoes, and more—and thus these women rarely need to make a concerted effort to ensure that their choline need is met.

If you focus on eating a balance of healthy foods, you're sure to get enough choline regardless of your genes. This is true not just for choline but for all nutrients. A diet that follows scientific guidelines concerning the types and amount of *foods* to eat, rather than the types and amounts of *nutrients*, will meet the nutrition needs of almost everyone regardless of genetic makeup. The government's MyPlate system and Marion Nestle's *What to Eat* guidelines, among others, tell *everyone* to eat more fruits and vegetables than anything else, to eat whole grains in preference to refined grains, to keep fried-food consumption at a minimum, and so forth. This general framework, which allows lots of room for individual choice, is the healthiest dietary framework for *all* human beings. Even when nutrigenomics gets to the point where patients can be given useful custom dietary recommendations based on genetic testing, no patient will ever be sent home with the advice to eat more fried foods than vegetables—or, for that matter, with the advice to eat one of Bill Wolcott's three diets based entirely on macronutrient proportions.

Know Thyself

The centerpiece of *The Metabolic Typing Diet* is a diagnostic questionnaire that was designed to help people increase their awareness about how different foods affect them and to identify their own metabolic type. I filled out this questionnaire when Wolcott's book was newly published. Having then recently reread a couple of my favorite books in Nietzsche's oeuvre, I had become so infatuated with the idea that maximum health (in the holistic Nietzschean sense) was life's true purpose that I decided to test the idea by trying to become as healthy as I possibly could in mind, body, and spirit in 100 days. I put a lot of effort into this project, selecting a special guide to help me pursue better health in each dimension of life, even going so far as to hire a psychotherapist to shore up my mental health (a story in itself). Wolcott was recommended to me as a possible dietary adviser. In the name of due diligence I read his book, which persuaded me to find a different diet mentor. The metabolic typing theory was a bit more (how shall I say?) *creative* than the kind of guidance I was looking for.

The questionnaire in particular left me scratching my head. It included lots of questions about the kinds of foods I most craved and enjoyed. When I got my result, it became evident that the test was grounded on the premise that the kinds of foods I most craved and enjoyed *defined* my metabolic type. Since most people base their diet on the foods they most crave and enjoy, it would seem that in the majority of cases this test would serve only to tell people to keep eating what they were already eating. Plus, most people have inherent weaknesses for "calorie bombs" such as refined grains, fatty meats, sweets, and fried foods, which are the very food types we can eat least of without screwing up our health. The idea that cravings were a reliable guide to the optimal personal diet seemed fundamentally unsound to me.

Despite this flaw, I liked Wolcott's general idea of using our experience of the effects of different foods on our physical and mental health to find the best-fitting personal diet. This was precisely how Friedrich Nietzsche settled upon the diet by which he attained his maximum of health.

It is a proven fact that people feel noticeably better when they follow healthy eating guidelines based on science. But within these guidelines, people have different experiences with specific foods and eating patterns. For example, some folks (myself included) feel terrific after drinking coffee and enjoy each day a little more when it begins with a mug of java. Others (like our friend Nietzsche) feel that coffee "spreads darkness" over their lives. Who knows which genes are involved? And who really needs to know? Nothing more than good old-fashioned self-awareness is required to identify such cause–effect patterns and make appropriate adjustments. Even the grossest errors of pleasure eating are correctible in this fashion. What sweet tooth doesn't feel awful after eating an entire pint of Ben & Jerry's after a full dinner?

And so, while we wait for nutritional genomics to mature to the point where it can help us fine-tune our individual diets within the one-size-fits-all parameters defined by science, it makes sense in the meantime to follow Nietzsche's example of paying attention to how different foods and eating patterns affect body and mind and tweaking our diet accordingly. I'd wager that even after the field of nutritional genomics is all grown up, people will still benefit from customizing their diet by feel to some extent. Science may never find a gene that explains why coffee makes some people feel good and others feel lousy, and I think I would continue to drink coffee—because of how I experience it—even if I was told I possessed a gene that kept me from getting any physical health benefit from it.

Discovering the optimal personal diet is a two-step process. Step one is to align your diet with the universal rules of healthy eating that science has defined. Step two is to experiment within this framework, paying close attention to how different foods and eating patterns affect you and adjusting them accordingly. There are a million and one different patterns you might observe. Perhaps cheese gives you headaches. Or maybe you have an easier time maintaining your weight when you eat fewer grains than the scientific guidelines permit. The possibilities are almost endless, and no expert outside of yourself can narrow them down for you.

My agnostic healthy-eating game—which, at last, I will fully describe in the next chapter—provides ideal conditions for pursuing one's optimal personal diet. It gets everyone started in the right place with a simple requirement to prioritize the food types that all humans need most of and to limit consumption of the food types that nobody can eat in large amounts without suffering consequences. Yet within this framework, there is plenty of room to come up with as idiosyncratic a dietary lifestyle as you like.

The psychological aspects of this process of developing your optimal personal diet—matters of taste, enjoyment, and identity—are no less important than the physical aspects. Remember, a person can function well physically on a wide range of diets. The ideal diet for any person is one that he not only functions well on but also really identifies with. Throughout this book, we have seen how important it is to identify with one's healthy diet, and all of the diet cults offer this potential. The agnostic healthy-eating game does too, but differently. First of all, it gives people an opportunity to choose a healthy way of eating that rejects the irrational priggishness of the One True Ways. But it also creates a space within which people may cultivate an individual dietary identity instead of completely submitting to a general doctrine, as in the healthy-diet cults. What's more, the loose framework of agnostic healthy-eating allows a person's eating identity to naturally evolve in response to changes in tastes and needs that are precipitated by aging and life experience, whereas the confining structure of most diet cults tends to thwart such evolution.

On the psychological level, this process is simply one of identifying particular ways of eating healthily that make you happy. Perhaps you will find happiness by throwing yourself into the art of cooking, mastering the most sophisticated recipes before going on to create original healthy meals worthy of a Michelin two-star rating. Or perhaps you will find happiness (and take pride) in figuring out how to eat healthily in the most environmentally responsible way possible. There are no wrong choices, as long as you stay within the framework of science-backed dietary guidelines and are happy.

The Benefits of Eating "Wrong"

It's possible that as you go through this process you will discover that a certain way of eating that makes you happy is technically less healthy than the way you've been eating. What should you do? Choose happiness. As long as the happier way of eating stays within the rules of agnostic healthy eating, you will come out ahead.

Consider the case of Steve Bratman. In the late 1970s, Bratman was a young hippie who lived in a commune in Upstate New York that occupied an organic farm. While he was there, he became an all-organic vegan who was so extreme in his quest for dietary purity that he tried to avoid eating anything that had been pulled out of the ground more than fifteen minutes earlier. This regimen made Bratman healthy enough physically, but it made him psychologically and socially unhealthy in equal measure. He ate each meal alone because he didn't want to be contaminated by contact with people who ate differently. He thought about food constantly and had a hard time talking about anything else. And for him, talking about food usually meant lecturing others on the One True Way to eat.

Over time, Bratman became increasingly aware of the price he was paying for his dietary perfectionism, and ultimately he abandoned his desultory path in favor of a low-fat, flexitarian, basically normal diet that made room for the occasional fast-food taco binge. He felt no worse physically on the new diet, and he was infinitely happier.

Bratman went on to earn a medical degree and to create a cottage industry of treating other obsessively healthy eaters and to pursue a mission of spreading awareness of the problem. In an essay published in the October 1997 issue of *Yoga Journal,* he coined the term "orthorexia nervosa" to indicate, as he described it, "an unhealthy obsession with healthy eating." Bratman wrote, "Orthorexia begins innocently enough, as a desire to overcome chronic illness or to improve general health. But because it requires considerable willpower to adopt a diet which differs radically from the food habits of childhood and the surrounding culture, few accomplish the change gracefully. Most must resort to an iron self-discipline bolstered by a hefty sense of superiority over those who eat junk food. Over time, what they eat, how much, and the consequences of dietary indiscretion come to occupy a greater and greater proportion of the orthorexic's day."

No doubt many of the yoga enthusiasts who read these words recognized themselves in them—which is not to say they accepted the diagnosis. To this day, Steve Bratman (who in 2001 published a book on orthorexia titled *Health Food Junkies*) receives hate mail from followers of various diet cults who accuse him of discouraging healthy eating. Of course, that's not what Bratman is really doing at all, but he does acknowledge the difficulty of advocating healthy eating without encouraging *obsessive* healthy eating. He wrote, "It often surprises me how blissfully unaware proponents of nutritional medicine remain of the propensity for their technique to create an obsession. Indeed, popular books on natural medicine seem to actively promote orthorexia in their enthusiasm for sweeping dietary changes."

The Key-in-Lock Myth

Underneath their differences, the modern healthy-diet cults share the belief that our bodies (particularly our genes) rigidly encode the exact diet that is required for maximum health, and that any mismatch between that code and what we actually eat will harm us. It's as if the body is a kind of lock and only one dietary key can open it to release optimal health. This concept overstates the truth and causes a good deal of needless anxiety. While not everyone is susceptible to the fear that this myth may inspire, there are more than a few men and women who, under its influence, become *desperate* to find the One True Way to nourish their genes and who dread the consequences of imperfection in their eating habits. Such anxiety is bad enough when a person assumes there is one perfect diet-genome match for all people, but how much worse is it for those who somehow are convinced that the dietary needs of individual humans are as unalike as those of different species!

If you are prone to this kind of anxiety, my advice to you is this: relax. Follow the example of our friend Nietzsche and think of your journey toward the optimal personal diet as an adventure of self-discovery and not as a frantic and hopeless effort to avoid all mistakes. Nietzsche never regretted the health struggles he had to surmount to fully become himself. He wasted no energy wishing away the bad luck of his migraines or the dietary missteps he learned from to develop the diet that made him healthiest and resonated with his sense of identity. For he discovered along the way that only through suffering and error is one able to discover and become oneself. Nietzsche captured this insight in his famous observation that "What does not kill us makes us stronger," an axiom that applies to diet as readily as it does to the rest of life, not in the sense that eating low-quality food makes us healthier but rather in the sense that, if we pay attention, eating "wrong" shows us how to eat "right" for ourselves. Believe me, as long as you're really trying, your dietary mistakes won't harm your physical health much and they will help you build a sense of identity around the way of eating that you develop, which is just as important.

A man who had an aphorism for every occasion, Nietzsche himself put it best: "Swallow your poison, for you need it badly."

15

Agnostic Healthy Eating

We have come to the final stop on our journey through and beyond the diet cults. Let's take a moment to review what we have seen on our myth-busting quest. It began at the beginning: taming fire, peopling the earth, the first human diets. We saw that the Journey of Man instilled in our species the ability to thrive on a wide variety of diets, from the high-fat diet of Crete to the high-carb diet of Hawaii to the high-protein diet of the Native Americans of northwest Montana. We learned that human beings are biologically adapted to cooked food, a fact that undercuts the diet cults' broadly shared conviction that it is unnatural and always unhealthy for people to "process" food. We saw, through the example of Paleo dieters, that people don't choose diets by reason; rather, diets choose people by appealing to identity-based dispositions such as masculine self-image. Later we saw (in connection with the bodybuilder's diet of protein and supplements) that people stay committed to their diet not so much because it "works" but because its rituals give them a sense of belonging.

In another series of loosely linked stops along our path, we saw that so-called superfoods such as blue-green algae are not really any better than ordinary foods and that demonized natural foods such as the potato are no worse. Nor are any of the individual nutrients that diet cults label good (water) or bad (sugar) truly good or bad in all amounts and contexts. We saw too that no diet is in itself sufficient to maximize health—that controlled and rational fasting and physical exercise make even the best diets better and may make a somewhat flawed diet good enough.

The remaining wayposts encountered in our travels exposed how the healthy-diet cults overemphasize the body and wrongly discount the mind and spirit. We saw that the secret to losing weight has little to do with what a person eats and everything to do with a person's mindset. We saw that eating and drinking for pleasure instead of health can be healthy nevertheless. We learned that the tendency of the healthy-diet cults to blame all disease on nutritional error is greatly overblown and distracts from other problems such as the epidemic of stress in the modern world. Finally, we saw that, contrary to diet-cult teachings, nutritional error can be useful in the process of developing a personal way of eating that not only maximizes physical health but also contributes to self-actualization—an objective of eating that the healthy-diet cults utterly fail to recognize.

The only conclusion we can draw from the sum of these lessons is that there is no such thing as the One True Way to eat for maximum health. No diet cult is better than the rest, and a person need not join any diet cult to attain maximum health. An agnostic approach to healthy eating that forbids nothing, smiles upon eating for pleasure, and encourages individual choice can do the job just as well or better.

Yet we've also seen that the healthy-diet cults often work very well for their followers. Bernie Freeman made a middle-age comeback as a raw-foodist. Brian MacKenzie improved his health, appearance, and performance on the Paleo Diet. Brandy Alles lost 100 pounds through Weight Watchers. John Romaniello sculpted a killer physique with the typical bodybuilder's menu of protein and supplements. Through their respective dietary conversions, these people attained a higher level of health than most people do outside of the diet cults. In each case the chosen diet supplied a doctrine to identify with and a community to belong to, making it easier to do the hard work of eating well enough to attain maximum health.

I hope that you are as covetous of the vitality of these folks as you are now convinced that diet cults are unnecessary to the attainment of maximum health. If so, then you are ready to learn about, and perhaps try, agnostic healthy eating. In this final chapter, I will describe a specific approach to agnostic healthy eating—a way to make a kind of game of it—that I developed for the sake of injecting into agnostic healthy eating some of the "stickiness" of the diet cults.

As I mentioned in Chapter 1, this game is defined by a single rule. This rule is based on, and fully consistent with, mainstream scientific guidelines for healthy eating that concern how often the various types of foods should be eaten. However, the game thus defined is simpler and more systematic than offerings such as the government's MyPlate program and, for this reason, easier to practice.

While my agnostic healthy-eating game has no basis in any of the several diet-cult myths discussed in the preceding chapters, it is a human invention and is shaped by the identity and experience of its inventor (me). No one can escape such biases in formulating opinions about how to eat. The best one can do is try to account for them. It is wise, therefore, to always "consider the source" when deciding whether to follow another person's dietary advice. With this idea in mind, I will preface my spiel on the agnostic healthy-eating game with a few words about where it came from.

Evolution of an Eater

Like most children of the 1970s (and before), I grew up on my mother's cooking. I was fortunate—Laurie enjoyed being in the kitchen and acquitted herself well with whisk and blade. Her early repertoire of dinner menus was cobbled together mainly from recipes she had learned from her own mother—standard fare such as meatloaf and spaghetti and meatballs, but better than my friends' mothers' meatloaf and spaghetti and meatballs.

When my brothers and I were small, our mom not only cooked like her mom but also thought as little about the nutritional quality of her cookery as her mother had. A teenager during the Great Depression, grandma knew the bitter ache of real hunger. So her idea of good nutrition was a full belly. Like many women who came of age in the Dust Bowl, she overcompensated a bit when raising the next generation in better times, and as a result her children struggled with their weight. Laurie's interest in nutrition began with a desire to keep off the fat she had lost in the fifth grade after the family physician put her on a diet (which, coming as it did from a mainstream medical professional, was agnostic, consisting of a few commonsense rules such as eating dessert only once a week).

Much later, when my brothers and I were in middle school, our mother developed a deeper interest in eating right, alongside millions of her fellow baby boomers then creeping toward middle age. We began to notice changes in the kinds of meals she prepared as well as in the sorts of packaged foods she brought home from the local Shop-n-Save. Our favorite sugary breakfast cereals (does anyone remember Kaboom! and King Vitamin?) gave way to blander alternatives such as Honey Nut Cheerios, homemade oatmeal (or "Fitz Porridge," as we liked to call our fruit-and-nut-rich version), and granola made from scratch. Laurie took out a subscription to *Bon Appétit* and began to test fancy new dishes from its pages on the family. Meatloaf and spaghetti and meatballs were replaced by things like white bean soup and broiled haddock with some kind of tomato-based Mediterranean-style sauce whose flavor remains sharp on my memory's tongue even though I haven't eaten it in twenty-five years.

I can't recall how my first ideas about good and bad nutrition formed. I do remember seeing a television commercial in the mid-1970s that boasted of a certain product's lack of cholesterol and asking my mom what cholesterol was. Her answer probably had something to do with heart attacks, which I would have understood because Laurie's father had already suffered one or two.

A few years later, when I was maybe nine years old, my mother instituted the practice of force-feeding her boys a spoonful of cod liver oil every morning before we left for school. When we asked her why we were being subjected to this strange torture, she said only that her mother had done the same to her. Nothing about omega fatty acids.

A fussy eater in my youth, I suppose I got much of my sense of good nutrition from the battles I had with my mother over eating vegetables.

Finish your spinach, Matthew.

I don't want to! It's gross!

I know you don't like it, honey, but it's good for you.

Predictably, when I left home for college my diet took a turn for the worse. By then I had quit running, so all those late-night pizzas and beers went straight to my love handles. Unable to muster the motivation to make better dietary choices, I slimmed down only when I started running again at the age of twenty-six.

Admittedly, my diet was somewhat improved by then, but not by much. At the very least, I was no longer living on pizza and beer. But there was still quite a bit of room for improvement. My typical lunch at that time was a typical lunch: a turkey sandwich with mayo on whole wheat bread, a small bag of potato chips, a glass of apple juice, and a cookie.

As I mentioned in Chapter 8, the cause of my getting back into running (and getting into triathlon) was my having stumbled into a career as an endurance sports writer. It was this same twist of fate that gave me the motivation to really clean up my diet. Through my work I developed a keen interest in sports nutrition. At first, this interest was limited to performance nutrition: sports drinks, supplements, and other things ingested specifically to boost speed and endurance in races. Eventually, though, my fascination with nutritional cause and effect broadened to encompass the general diet.

By the time I earned a professional certification in sports nutrition in 2006, I had long since elevated my own dietary standards to the level they remain at today. Most of the changes I made were based on things I had known since I was a child and on an intuitive sense that agnostic healthy eating was the right way to go. Since kindergarten, for example, I had known that fruits and vegetables were healthy and that one ought to eat lots of them. So I ate more fruits and vegetables. For almost my entire life, too, I had known that it is not healthy to eat sweets in large amounts. So I ate fewer sweets. I did not eliminate any foods from my diet or seek out specific foods to add to it but simply shifted the balance of foods in my diet toward those of higher quality. In other words, I became an agnostic healthy eater.

Nothing I learned in my nutritional education contradicted my childhood knowledge or dietary intuitions. The mainstream science that I chose to base my education on clearly confirmed that an inclusive, flexible, high-quality diet sufficed to support optimal health. Further confirmation came from my exposure to world-class endurance athletes, the vast majority of whom attain the highest degree of health possible through agnostic healthy eating.

Of course, like everyone else I was also exposed to the recruitment efforts of advocates for low-fat, low-carb, high-protein, Zone, vegan, probiotic, macrobiotic, Paleo, Chinese, Mediterranean, gluten-free, food-combining, portion-control, low-glycemic, raw, alkaline, detox, and high-starch diet cults, among others. But I could not take these people seriously. They seemed to me like so many carnival barkers, aiming for persuasion rather than truth. Indeed, it was incredible to me that *anyone* could fall for the "Hear ye, hear ye" of these hucksters with so few real scientists among them and so many scientists endorsing (at least implicitly) the agnostic way. I have since discovered that there are indeed many others who are equally turned off by diet-cult dogma, but that, unfortunately, most of these folks don't see a compelling alternative in agnostic healthy eating.

I thought that perhaps the agnostic approach to healthy eating just needed a message makeover. In my 2009 book *Racing Weight,* I tried to do my part, turning the shtick-free high-quality diet I now shared with many top endurance athletes into a game that other athletes could use to maximize their general health and fitness. In it, I unveiled the Diet Quality Score, a tool that separated foods into ten categories. Six were labeled high-quality foods and four were labeled low-quality foods. Eating a high-quality food added points to an athlete's daily Diet Quality Score, whereas eating a low-quality food subtracted points. The maximum possible daily DQS was thirty-two points. I did not tell my readers that they had to score thirty-two points every day—or any day, for that matter. I just encouraged them to raise their score until they got the results they sought.

A few years later, I modified this game to make it even simpler. In the new version, I created a diet-quality hierarchy that ranked the ten categories of food by quality and instructed athletes to simply eat each food type more often than any type of lesser quality (with some flexibility). This one rule was designed to ensure that overall diet quality was high enough to maximize health and performance while allowing freedom to eat everything, to eat for pleasure, and to exercise individual preferences. I was fully aware that my rule was arbitrary in the sense that one could easily come up with other specific guidelines for healthy eating that yielded the same results. But you would be hard pressed to come up with an agnostic healthy eating game that was more elegantly simple, hence more practical or sustainable for people with a wide range of lifestyles and budgets.

Although I created the agnostic healthy-eating game for endurance athletes, its usefulness is not limited to that population. Anyone can play it, and if enough people do, a community of agnostic healthy eaters will be born, and thereafter it will be much easier for folks who can't stomach (so to speak) the One True Ways to find an alternative that gives them everything they want out of their diet.

The Diet Quality Hierarchy

There is more than one way to categorize foods by basic type. I don't doubt that a degree of cultural and temporal bias exists in the way I've chosen to do it. A nutritionist in Thailand might have done it somewhat differently, and the list drawn up by someone living two hundred years ago or two hundred years from now might be different still. But I think my list is sensible for here and now. The ten categories of foods in my agnostic healthy-eating game are, in decreasing order of quality:

- vegetables
- fruits

- nuts, seeds, and healthy oils
- high-quality meat and seafood
- whole grains
- dairy
- refined grains
- low-quality meat and seafood
- sweets
- fried foods

The first two foods in this hierarchy are classified as *essential* foods. This means that they are required in the agnostic healthy-eating game and are to be eaten more often than any other food type. While I encourage you to eat veggies more often than fruits, this isn't essential. The reason vegetables and fruits are classified as essential is that science has plainly shown that they must be eaten in abundance for maximum health to be attained.

The next four food types in the hierarchy—nuts, seeds, and healthy oils; high-quality meat and seafood; whole grains; and dairy—are classified as *recommended* foods. This means you don't have to eat them, but you should unless you have a compelling reason not to (such as ethical qualms about eating meat or a peanut allergy), because science has shown that health tends to improve when each of these food types is added to the diet. All of the "recommended" food types should be eaten more often than any of the foods in the "acceptable" food class. How often you eat each in relation to the others in the "recommended" food class is up to you (science doesn't tell us whether it's healthier to eat nuts, seeds, and healthy oils more often than whole grains or vice versa), but balancing them according to their order in the hierarchy is a good place to start.

Refined grains, low-quality meat and seafood, sweets, and fried foods are classified as *acceptable* foods. You can eat them in small amounts without negative consequences, but science shows that when any of them is eaten in large amounts, health takes a hit. Therefore each is to be eaten less often than any food type in the other classes. Ideally, you will eat the lowest-quality foods within this class least often.

So the one rule of the agnostic healthy eating game is this: on a weekly basis, eat each type of "essential" food more often than any type of "recommended" food, and eat each type of "recommended" food more often than any type of "acceptable" food. For extra credit, eat each of the ten food types in the diet-quality hierarchy more often than any food type of lower rank. This rule does not represent the One True Way to eat for maximum health, but if you heed it (and get plenty of exercise) you will be as physically healthy as you can be, and if you take full advantage of its intrinsic flexibility you will also enjoy eating and will cultivate a personal eating identity that makes you happy.

To play the agnostic healthy-eating game, simply keep a record of everything you eat by food type for one week and aim to be in obedience to the one rule by the end of the week. It doesn't matter if you are out of balance in one meal or even one full day, as long as you are in balance by week's end. Before I share the finer points of the agnostic healthy-eating game, let me say a few words about the reasoning behind the ordering of food types in the diet-quality hierarchy.

Essential Foods

Let's first take a closer look at the two essential foods in the diet-quality hierarchy.

Vegetables

Scientific support for the mainstream recommendation to eat a lot of vegetables (greens, root vegetables, legumes, etc.) is about as rock-solid as the evidence that seatbelts and air bags in cars save lives. Eating a lot of vegetables is arguably the single best thing you can do for your health. Those who eat the most vegetables have a reduced risk for a long list of chronic diseases, they look and feel better, and they live much longer than those who eat the fewest veggies.

A person who pays little attention to nutrition except when a new diet study is mentioned on the local television news might assume that no diet cult is barmy enough to brand vegetables a forbidden food, but that assumption would be wrong. Fruitarians eat no vegetables. None. Some low-carb diets forbid "starchy" vegetables such as potatoes. Many Paleo dieters avoid legumes. And men and women on anti-inflammation diets often avoid nightshade vegetables such as eggplant.

Fruits

Fruits (berries, tropical fruits, apples, etc.) have the same beneficial health effects as vegetables. However, research suggests that the two food types achieve these effects in somewhat different ways because their nutrient profiles are complementary and synergistic. That's why both are classified as essential. I rank fruit lower than vegetables in quality only because vegetable nutrition is somewhat more diverse.

As foolish as it may seem, there are diet cults that either forbid or strictly limit fruit intake. Fruit is acceptable only as an occasional treat in certain low-sugar diets. Some hard-core Paleo dieters also eat little or no fruit. The problem that many people seem to have with fruit is that it contains fructose. Research indicates that eating large amounts of *processed* foods and beverages containing lots of *added* fructose from *refined* sources is associated with negative health outcomes. Lumping fruit together with such sweets under the label "unhealthy" because they both contain fructose is like lumping meat together with certain types of bombs under the label "dangerous explosives" because they both contain nitrogen.

Recommended Foods

You don't have to eat the four foods in the "recommended" class, but I would if I were you, and here's why.

Nuts, Seeds, and Healthy Oils

People who eat lots of nuts and seeds have a lower risk of heart disease than do people who seldom eat these foods. They also live longer. A massive epidemiological study published in 2013 found that men and women who ate nuts every day were 20 percent less likely to die over a thirty-year period than were those who ate no nuts. Yet nuts and seeds are forbidden or restricted in some low-fat diets, such as Dean Ornish's. The reason is, of course, that nuts and seeds are high in fat, which makes people fat and increases the risk of heart disease. Except it doesn't—at least not when it comes from nuts and seeds.

I group healthy oils together with nuts and seeds because they are similar in both nutrition and benefits—indeed, they often come from the same source. Healthy oils are defined as all non-fried plant oils extracted by non-chemical means. Examples are coconut oil, olive oil, and peanut oil.

I think it's possible to be very healthy without nuts, seeds, and healthy oils in the diet, but it's easier with them. They are rich in the fats and proteins that fruits and vegetables generally lack. They would be a poor substitute for fruits and vegetables, though, because they can't match the dazzling array of micronutrients that the two higher-quality food categories have.

High-Quality Meats and Seafood

This category includes most wild-caught fish and shellfish, only the highest-quality farm-raised seafood, the leanest meat cuts, and meats from wild game and free-ranging animals fed natural diets. Lots of studies have shown that eating fish (and other seafood) is healthy. Frequent fish consumption slows down brain aging, for example. Eating lots of meat, on the other hand, is generally associated with less-favorable health outcomes. But I think that's because most of the meat that is eaten today is of low quality. Meat from free-ranging animals raised on natural diets is almost certainly just as healthy as wild-caught fish. Meat has been a significant component of human and human-ancestor diets for millions of years. Eaten selectively and in moderation, it can't possibly be bad for us in any meaningful sense of "bad."

As we know, lots of people are convinced that eating meat and fish in any amount is unhealthy. Colin Campbell, author of *The China Study*, is one of the most prominent experts who believe that animal flesh should be rigidly excluded from the diet. But such voices are greatly outnumbered by those in the nutrition-science mainstream who say that moderate amounts of fish and high-quality meat in the diet are healthy.

What we need is a good epidemiological study that distinguishes discriminating meat-eaters (who eat mostly organic meats, meats from animals fed natural diets, meats from free-ranging animals, lean cuts of meat, and not too much meat overall) from indiscriminate meat eaters (who eat large amounts of industrially produced, fatty, and processed meats). I am confident such a study would find that eaters of high-quality meat are at least as healthy as vegetarians. In the meantime, it is enough for me to know that most of the world's healthiest group of people, elite endurance athletes, eat meat and fish.

It's worth noting that studies have generally found that eating eggs (which I include in this category) is associated with favorable health outcomes. According to one study, eating two eggs for breakfast is good for your waistline. The only real difference between eggs and meat, as between fish and meat, is that eggs tend to be closer to their natural form than is much of the meat that is eaten today.

Whole Grains

Whole grains (whole wheat, brown rice, oats, etc.) contain more carbohydrate than anything else. Carbohydrates have one main purpose in the body: providing short-term energy. The amount of carbohydrate that a person needs is determined by his activity level. A couch potato should not eat a lot of whole grains, while a cyclist might have a hard time getting enough carbs without eating whole grains at least a couple of times a day. So while whole grains are ranked fifth in the diet-quality hierarchy, extremely active people should feel free to eat them more often than any of the other food types in the "recommended" class.

Grains are forbidden and restricted in a growing list of diet cults including the Paleo Diet and gluten-free diets. Followers of these diets accuse grains of causing systemic inflammation and other problems, even in the absence of conditions such as celiac disease. Research has shown that the people who eat the most whole grains actually have *lower* levels of systemic inflammation plus a reduced risk of developing cardiovascular disease.

Dairy

Anyone can get by without dairy (milk, yogurt, cheese, cream, etc.) in the diet, and the two adults out of every three who are lactose-intolerant are better off avoiding non-fermented dairy foods. Plenty of diet cults either outlaw dairy (vegan, Paleo) or restrict it (low-fat). Yet health science has been kind to dairy. In 2010 a major review of past research, authored by British scientists, reported that the subjects who consumed the most dairy products had a lower risk of heart disease, stroke, diabetes, and "all-cause mortality" than did those who ate the least dairy.

On balance, dairy deserves a spot as the lowest-ranked among the recommended foods, which again are foods that you should include in your diet unless you have a good reason not to (such as lactose intolerance).

Acceptable Foods

Now let's take a closer look at the four "acceptable" food types in the diet quality hierarchy.

Refined Grains

I classify refined grains (white flour, white rice, etc.) as a merely acceptable food because they are significantly less healthful than the whole grains they are made from. With so many whole-grain versions of popular foods to choose from—including whole-grain breakfast cereals, breads, and pastas—there is little need to include many refined grains in one's diet.

It certainly won't harm you to eat a plate of pasta made the traditional way at a fine Italian restaurant for the sake of a more pleasurable eating experience. I merely recommend eating refined grains less often than you eat any of the six higher-quality food types.

Low-Quality Meats and Seafood

This category includes all processed meats and all but the leanest cuts of unprocessed meats. These foods have a lot of good stuff in them, but research has shown quite clearly that it is best not to eat them in large amounts. The category also includes farm-raised seafood that does not meet the quality standards of watchdog organizations such as the Aquaculture Stewardship Council.

Like refined grains, low-quality meat and seafood is a food type that is made largely unnecessary in the diet—even the meat-lover's diet—by a high-quality alternative: in this case, high-quality meat and seafood. I wouldn't want to live in a world without bacon, but the totality of evidence suggests that low-quality meats should be consumed less often than the "essential" and "recommended" food types and probably less often than refined grains as well.

Sweets

In the right circumstances (say, insulin shock) a slice of German chocolate cake could save your life. Sweets are not intrinsically bad and refined sugar is not poison by any sane definition. Even the most unrepentant sweet tooth cannot deny, however, that sweets (soft drinks, candy, desserts, etc.) have a lower "threshold of excess" than almost any other category of food. As I mentioned in Chapter 10, people who drink several soft drinks each day or the equivalent are far more likely than is the average person to become overweight and diabetic and to develop heart disease. If you want to look great naked and be as healthy on the inside as you look on the outside, then you should eat sweets less often than any other type of food—except fried foods.

Fried Foods

It's a shame that fried foods (snack chips, french fries, fried chicken, donuts, etc.) are so delicious, because a person cannot eat them in more than minimal amounts without suffering negative consequences. Research has consistently shown that fried foods are among the few specific foods that fat people eat more often than normal-weight individuals. Frying also generates carcinogens known as aldehydes. One study found that female rats fed a potato chip-supplemented diet produced offspring with neural and muscular defects.

I try to eat fried foods less often than all other food types, and I think that's a good idea for anyone who wishes to be very healthy.

Forbidden Foods

Oh, wait a minute: There are no forbidden foods in agnostic healthy eating.

There is, however, a catch-all "Other Foods" category for certain foods and food-like things that don't fit in the ten main categories just described. Most sauces, condiments, and dressings, most energy and snack bars, and many highly processed foods made from originally healthy foods (e.g., rice milk) should be counted as other foods, which are classified as "acceptable."

Diet Quality Hierarchy/Agnostic Healthy-Eating Game Cheat Sheet

The following table summarizes the important points of the diet quality hierarchy as it relates to the agnostic healthy-eating game.

Type	Rank	Classification	Examples	Guidelines
Vegetables	1	Essential	Raw vegetables Cooked vegetables Salads Vegetable soups and purees Vegetable juices	Ideally: Eat more often than any other food type Minimally: Eat more often than anything except fruit
Fruits	2	Essential	Whole fruits Stewed fruits Applesauce Fruit smoothies 100% fruit spreads 100% fruit juices	Ideally: Eat more often than anything except vegetables Minimally: Same as Ideally
Nuts, Seeds, and Healthy Oils	3	Recommended	Peanuts (technically a legume), almonds, cashews, pine nuts, macadamia nuts, sunflower seeds, chia seeds, hemp seeds Nut butters (without sugar) Plant oils produced without chemical extractions	Ideally: Eat more often than anything except vegetables and fruit Minimally: Eat more often than any food type in the Acceptable category

High-Quality Meats and Seafood	4	Recommended	Meat from grass-fed and free-range animals Organic meats Meats with less than 10% fat All fish Eggs	Ideally: Eat more often than anything except vegetables, fruits, and nuts, seeds, and healthy oils Minimally: Eat more often than any food type in the Acceptable category
Whole Grains	5	Recommended	Whole wheat, oats, barley, corn, brown rice, teff, amaranth, quinoa 100% whole-grain breads 100% whole-grain breakfast cereals 100% whole-grain pastas	Ideally: Eat more often than all low-quality food types and dairy Minimally: Eat more often than any food type in the Acceptable category
Dairy	6	Recommended	Whole, reduced-fat, and skim milk from cows, goats, and sheep Cheese Yogurt without added sugar Sour cream Cream cheese	Ideally: Eat more often than any food type in the Acceptable category Minimally: Same as Ideally
Refined Grains	7	Acceptable	Refined or enriched wheat flour White rice Breads made with less than 100% whole grains Breakfast cereals made with less than 100% whole grains Pastas made with less than 100% whole grains	Ideally: Eat less often than anything except low-quality meats, sweets, and fried foods Minimally: Eat less often than any food in the Essential and Recommended categories
Low-Quality Meats and Seafood	8	Acceptable	Most cold cuts Most processed meats (e.g., bacon) All meats that do not qualify as high-quality	Ideally: Eat less often than anything except sweets and fried foods Minimally: Eat less often than any food in the Essential and Recommended categories

| Sweets | 9 | Acceptable | Candy
Pastries
Desserts
Soft drinks
Diet soft drinks
Most energy bars
Some breakfast cereals | Ideally: Eat less often than anything except fried foods

Minimally: Eat less often than any food in the Essential and Recommended categories |
| Fried Foods | 10 | Acceptable | Snack chips
French fries
Fried chicken
Donuts | Ideally: Eat less often than any other food type

Minimally: Eat less often than any food in the Essential and Recommended categories |

Playing the Game

The agnostic healthy-eating game is based entirely on the frequency with which different types of foods are eaten. When you begin to play this game, you will immediately confront the question of what constitutes an "occasion" of eating a particular type of food. Instead of relying on official serving sizes defined by the government or by product labels, I suggest you think in terms of normal portion sizes for you. Examples of normal portion sizes for most people are one cup of cooked vegetables, a whole piece of fruit, a small handful of nuts or seeds, a palm-size serving of meat or fish, two slices of bread, and an eight-ounce tub of yogurt.

Some servings should be counted as double or half portions. For example, I would count the onions, tomatoes, and mushrooms in an omelet as a half portion of vegetables (even though mushrooms are technically a fungus). A thirty-two-ounce soda I would count as two sweets.

Composite foods can be even trickier. How do you handle a few slices of pizza with pepperoni and olives? Use common sense to make these calls. The pizza crust I'd count as a refined grain, the tomato sauce and olives combined as a half portion of vegetables, the cheese as dairy, and the pepperoni as a low-quality meat.

This isn't science. It's just a science-backed tool for eating well. God has no opinion about how your chicken burrito with rice, pinto beans, lettuce, guacamole, jack cheese, and salsa should be categorized. Figure it out for yourself, with the general guidelines I've provided and your common sense. See Appendix A for detailed instructions on classifying foods in the agnostic healthy-eating game.

You may have noticed that my game has no rules concerning the overall amount of food that is eaten. This is because you can trust your appetite to ensure that you do not generally overeat if you are obeying the game's one hard-and-fast rule and getting plenty of aerobic exercise.

You do not need to play the agnostic healthy-eating game every single week for the rest of your life. I myself played the game originally only long enough to get it right. Nowadays I conduct periodic dietary audits, where I resume the game for one week here and there just to make sure I'm not slipping. Once you have your diet dialed in, I suggest you transition to periodic audits as well.

Appendix B presents a sample scoring sheet that you can use to play the agnostic healthy-eating game. Appendix C offers an example of a typical week of agnostic healthy eating as I practice it. Take it as a template, not a blueprint. You could play the game just as faithfully as I do with a totally different set of meals and snacks. Remember, it is companions I seek, not followers.

Appendix A

Following are detailed guidelines for categorizing foods when playing the agnostic healthy-eating game.

Vegetables

This category includes whole, fresh vegetables eaten raw or cooked as well as canned and frozen vegetables and pureed or liquefied vegetables used in soups, sauces, and so forth. Legumes (peas, lentils, etc.) are also counted as vegetables.

Vegetable juices may be counted as a portion of vegetables once per day.

Fruits that are generally regarded as vegetables for culinary purposes— including tomatoes and avocados—may be counted as vegetables.

A composite food containing more than one type of vegetable may be counted as 1.5 or 2 servings of vegetables.

Generous amounts of vegetables on a sandwich may be counted as ½ portion of vegetables. A little iceberg lettuce and a thin, pink tomato slice on a hamburger should not be counted at all.

Non-fried vegetable snack chips such as kale chips may be counted as ½ portion of vegetables one time per day.

Plant-based powdered supplements such as Greens Plus also may be counted as ½ portion of vegetables one time per day.

Tofu and other lightly processed soy products as well as other lightly processed foods made entirely or almost entirely from vegetables should be counted as ½ serving of vegetables.

Spinach pasta and spinach tortillas should not be scored as vegetables. They should be counted as refined grains.

Typical serving sizes of vegetables include a fist-size portion of solid vegetables, ½ cup of tomato sauce, and a medium-size bowl of vegetable soup or salad.

Fruit

This category includes whole fresh fruits, canned and frozen fruits, cooked whole fruits, blended fruits, dried fruits, and foods made with whole fruits, such as applesauce.

Small amounts of fruit included in baked goods, packaged yogurt, etc. should not be counted at all.

One-hundred percent fruit juice should be counted as ½ portion of fruit. Juice products that are less than 100 percent fruit juice and contain added sugars should be counted as sweets.

Fruit-based desserts such as peach cobbler may be double-scored as fruits and sweets.

Fruit-based products such as dried cranberries and applesauce that contain added sugar should be double-scored as fruits and sweets.

All processed-fruit snacks such as Fruit Rollups should be counted as sweets.

Foods that include multiple fruits, such as smoothies, may be counted as 1.5 to 2 servings of fruit.

Fruits such as tomatoes and avocados that are treated as vegetables in culinary tradition should be counted as vegetables.

Typical serving sizes of fruits include one medium-size piece of whole fruit (e.g., one banana), a handful of berries, and ½ cup of applesauce.

Nuts, Seeds, and Healthy Oils

This category includes cashews, almonds, walnuts, sunflower seeds, hempseeds, etc. Peanuts should be counted as nuts although they are technically legumes.

This category also includes non-chemically extracted plant oils consumed raw or cooked in small amounts. For example, an olive oil-based dressing on a salad is to be counted as a serving of healthy oil, as is grapeseed oil used to sauté vegetables.

Nut and seed butters made without sugar or other additives besides salt should be counted as nuts, seeds, and healthy oils. Those made with added sugar should be counted as sweets.

Typical serving sizes of nuts, seeds, and healthy oils include a handful of nuts, enough peanut butter to cover a slice of toast, and two tablespoons of salad dressing.

High-Quality Meats and Seafood

This category includes all meat from wild game (venison, pheasant, etc.), free-range fowl and poultry, and grass-fed cattle and lamb.

This category also includes non-processed lean cuts from non-wild/free range/grass-fed animals, as in these examples:

Beef
Eye of round, filet mignon, London broil, round roast, sirloin tip side steak, top round roast/steak, top sirloin, and 90 percent-plus lean ground beef

Chicken
All parts except skin and organs

Lamb
Lamb shoulder, leg of lamb, loin chops

Pork
Canadian-style bacon, extra-lean ham, loin roast, loin chop, tenderloin

Turkey
All parts except skin and organs

All forms of *wild-caught* fresh, frozen, and canned fish and shellfish are included in this category except American eel, Atlantic salmon (both wild and farmed), imported catfish, and imported shrimp (for reasons of contamination).

All products carrying the Marine Stewardship Council's "Fish Forever" label are to be counted as high-quality seafood.

Only those *farmed* seafood products that bear the Aquaculture Stewardship Council's "Responsibly Farmed" consumer label may be counted as high-quality seafood.

Typical serving sizes of high-quality meat and seafood include one hamburger patty and a palm-size piece of fish.

Whole Grains
This category includes whole wheat, buckwheat, barley, brown rice, corn, oats, amaranth, quinoa, spelt, bulgur, millet, rye, sorghum, and teff.

The whole-grains category also includes breads and other baked goods, pastas, and breakfast cereals made with 100-percent whole grains and no refined grains.

Whole-bean flours such as garbanzo bean flour may be counted as whole grains even though, technically, they are processed legumes.

Homemade popcorn counts as a whole grain. (Movie-theater popcorn, microwave popcorn, and bagged, ready-to-eat popcorn do not.)

Typical serving sizes of whole-grain foods include two slices of bread and a medium-size bowl of breakfast cereal.

Dairy
This category includes cow's milk, goat's milk, sheep's milk, cheese, yogurt, sour cream, cream cheese, cottage cheese, and butter.

Whole milk, low-fat milk, and skim milk products are all counted as dairy, but whole-milk dairy products are preferable.

All sweetened dairy products, including ice cream, frozen yogurt, sweet cream, chocolate milk, and yogurts containing some form of sugar as their second ingredient should be counted as sweets.

All "fake" milk and cheese products (soy milk, rice milk, tofu cheese, etc.) should be placed in the "Other Foods" category.

Typical serving sizes of dairy foods include the amount of milk you would normally use in a bowl of breakfast cereal, two slices of deli cheese, and a single-serving tub of yogurt.

Refined Grains
This category includes white rice, processed flours, and all breakfast cereals, pastas, breads, and other baked goods made with less than 100-percent whole grains.

Note that, in wheat-containing products, any description other than "whole wheat," "whole wheat flour," or "whole grain wheat flour" indicates that the wheat is refined and the product should be counted as a refined grain.

Breakfast cereals containing more than 10 grams of sugar per serving should be counted as sweets, unless they contain dried fruit.

Whole-grain baked goods should be counted as sweets if they contain enough sugar to taste sweet.

Typical serving sizes of refined grains include a fist-size portion of white rice, a medium-size bowl of pasta or breakfast cereal, and two slices of bread.

Other Foods

This category includes all condiments, sauces, and gravies except those that are made from high-quality foods, such as guacamole, hummus, mustard, pesto, and salsa, which may be scored as ½ portion of the food type they belong to. For example, salsa may be scored as ½ portion of vegetables.

Beer, wine, and spirits after the first drink of the day should be counted as other Foods. The first drink should not be counted at all. Mixed drinks containing sugar should be counted as sweets.

Energy and snack bars are to be counted as other foods unless they are made exclusively from high-quality foods such as whole grains, nuts, and seeds.

This category also includes all processed fake dairy products and meats such as rice milk and tofu burgers.

All nutritional supplements including protein powders and meal replacements should be counted as other foods, except for plant-based powder supplements such as Greens Plus, which may be counted as ½ portion of vegetables one time per day.

Low-Quality Meats and Seafood

This category includes all meats and seafoods that are not included in the high-quality meat and fish category.

All processed meats (sausage, most cold cuts, bacon, jerky, cured meats, hot dogs, chicken nuggets, etc.) should be counted as low-quality.

All red meat contained in packaged products or eaten at restaurants should be counted as low-quality unless you have specific knowledge that it came from a wild or grass-fed animal or is at least 90 percent lean.

Always count farm-raised seafoods as low-quality unless they bear the Aquaculture Stewardship Council's "Responsibly Farmed" consumer label.

Animal fats used for cooking, including bacon grease and lard, should be counted as low-quality meats.

Typical serving sizes of low-quality meat and seafood include one hamburger patty and a palm-size piece of fish.

Sweets
This category includes all foods and beverages containing substantial amounts of refined sugars, including soft drinks, candy, pastries, and other desserts.

All food and beverages sweetened artificially should be considered sweets.

Honey, maple syrup, and agave nectar are not counted as sweets. Don't count them at all.

Coffee drinks sweetened with sugar or dairy should be categorized as sweets.

Dark chocolate does not count as a sweet if it's at least 80 percent cacao and consumed in small amounts of 100 calories or less.

Breakfast cereals with more than 10 grams of sugar per serving are to be considered sweets unless they contain dried fruit.

All fruit juices containing added sugar and all processed fruit snacks such as Fruit Rollups should be counted as sweets.

Yogurt products containing some form of sugar as their second ingredient should be counted as sweets.

Typical serving sizes of sweets include a slice of pie, a small candy bar, and a 12-ounce can of soda.

Fried Foods
This category includes all deep-fried foods such as potato chips, fried chicken, fritters, and donuts.

Pan-fried, stir-fried, and sautéed foods do not count as fried foods.

Typical serving sizes of fried foods include a small bag of potato chips and one whole donut.

Appendix B

Use this table to keep track of how often you eat foods of each type during one week. Use lines to represent one occasion of eating a given type of food. Use vertical lines to indicate full portions and dots to indicate half-portions.

Food Type	Number of Times Eaten This Week
Vegetables	
Fruit	
Nuts and Seeds	
Fish and High-Quality Meats	
Whole Grains	
Dairy	
Refined Grains	
Other Foods	
Low-Quality Meats	
Sweets	
Fried Foods	

Appendix C

While I was writing this book, I played my own agnostic healthy-eating game for one week. Here I share my record of what I ate (and drank) on those seven days not for prescriptive purposes but merely to give you a concrete example of the game in action.

Monday

You will see a lot of peaches in this food journal. That's because my wife and I have a peach tree in our back yard and it was bearing fruit at the time I recorded this journal. There's nothing wrong with eating what you have!

Breakfast	
Bowl of Life breakfast cereal with whole milk and blueberries	1 Whole grain
	1 Dairy
Orange juice	2 Fruits
Coffee	
Lunch	
Brown rice, bean, and vegetable burrito with whole-wheat tortilla and tomato salsa	2 Whole grains
	3 Vegetables
Butternut squash soup	1 Fruit
Spicy Hot V8 juice	
Peach	
Snack	
Almonds	1 Nuts, seeds, and healthy oils
Dinner	
Pork tenderloin	1 High-quality meat and seafood
Mixed vegetables	1 Vegetable
Toasted whole-wheat bread with old-fashioned peanut butter	1 Whole grain
	1 Nuts, seeds, and healthy oils
Beer	
Dark chocolate	
Snack	
Peach	1 Fruit

Tuesday

If it seems like I eat a lot of food, that's because I do. Because I exercise at least 90 minutes a day I need to consume eat least 3,000 calories a day to avoid wasting away.

Breakfast Bowl of Grape Nuts Flakes breakfast cereal with whole milk and blueberries Orange juice Coffee	1 Whole grain 1 Dairy 2 Fruits
Lunch Leftover pork tenderloin Leftover mixed vegetables Toasted whole-wheat bread with old- fashioned peanut butter Spicy Hot V8 juice Peach	1 High-quality meat and seafood 2 Vegetables 1 Whole grain 1 Nuts, seeds, and healthy oils 1 Fruit
Snack Cashews	1 Nuts, seeds, and healthy oils
Dinner Baked tilapia Boiled potatoes with olive oil, salt, and pepper Brussels sprouts 2 beers Dark chocolate	1 High-quality meat and seafood 2 Vegetables 1 Other (2nd beer)
Snack Greek yogurt (whole milk) with dried cherries, honey, and Grape Nuts Flakes	1 Dairy ½ Fruit ½ Whole grain

Wednesday

I went out for lunch with my wife on this particular day. The restaurant we selected served no whole-grain breads, so I got my sandwich on ciabatta bread and enjoyed every bite of it. We were still away from home when I got hungry again and ducked inside a Starbucks for a pumpkin muffin. That's two refined grains in one day—but they were the only two refined grains I ate all week.

Breakfast	
Bowl of Life breakfast cereal with whole milk	1 Whole grain
and blueberries	1 Dairy
Orange juice	2 Fruits
Coffee	
Lunch	
Grilled vegetable sandwich with cheese on	1 Vegetable
ciabatta bread	1 Refined grain
Fruit smoothie	1 Fruit
	1 Dairy (cheese + yogurt in smoothie)
Snack	
Pumpkin muffin	1 Refined grain
Dinner	
Grilled marinated chicken breasts	1 High-quality meat and seafood
Brussels sprouts	1 Vegetable
Whole-wheat toast with old-fashioned peanut	1 Whole grain
butter	1 Nuts, seeds, and healthy oils
Beer	
Dark chocolate	
Snack	
Peach	1 Fruit

Thursday

Perhaps you have noticed that there is a lot of repetition in my diet. I eat more or less the same breakfast every day, I rely on Spicy Hot V8 juice to provide an extra vegetable portion at lunch, and so forth. These habits are elements of the eating identity I have developed.

Breakfast	
Bowl of Grape Nuts Flakes breakfast cereal	1 Whole grain
with whole milk and blueberries	1 Dairy
Orange juice	2 Fruits
Coffee	
Snack	
Fruit smoothie	2 Fruits
Lunch	
Chicken Caesar salad	2 Vegetables
Spicy Hot V8 juice	1 High-quality meat and seafood
	1 Other (Caesar dressing)
Snack	
Almonds	1 Nuts, seeds, and healthy oils
Dinner	
Tuna casserole with whole-wheat pasta and	2 Vegetables
peas	1 High-quality meat and seafood
Small Caesar salad	1 Whole grain
Beer	
Dark chocolate	
Snack	
Greek yogurt (whole milk) with dried	1 Dairy
cherries, honey, and Grape Nuts Flakes	½ Fruit
	½ Whole grain

Friday

I drank three alcoholic beverages on the evening of this day, which almost qualifies as a binge. This is not unusual for me. I like to drink and typically relax my one-drink limit one night a week. One of the things I like about the agnostic healthy-eating game is that it affords freedom to indulge personal dietary weaknesses to a harmless extent by assigning a general limit to consumption of lower-quality (i.e. "acceptable") foods and allowing the individual to balance the food types within this classification against one another. I eat fewer sweets and fried foods so I can drink more beer, but someone else might consume less alcohol and eat fewer low-quality meats so she can eat more sweets.

Breakfast	
Bowl of Life breakfast cereal with whole milk and blueberries	1 Whole grain
	1 Dairy
Orange juice	2 Fruits
Coffee	
Lunch	
Leftover tuna casserole with whole-wheat pasta and peas	2 Vegetables
	1 Whole grain
Spicy Hot V8 juice	1 High-quality meat and seafood
Snack	
Cashews	1 Nuts, seeds, and healthy oils
Beer	
Dinner	
Oysters Rockefeller	2 High-quality meat and seafood
Beet salad	3 Vegetables
Filet mignon	4 Other (wine and sauces)
Mashed potatoes	1 Sweet
Spring peas	
2 glasses wine	
Cheesecake	

Saturday

As you see, I make a regular habit of eating dinner leftovers for lunch. It's convenient for me because I work at home, so I don't have to worry about packaging leftovers to take to the office. I've also found that it's easier to work vegetables into my lunches with leftovers than it is with traditional lunch fare such as sandwiches.

Breakfast	
Whole-wheat bagel with cream cheese, lox, red onions, tomato, and capers	1 Whole grain 1 Dairy
Orange juice	1 High-quality meat and seafood
Coffee	1 Fruit
	½ Vegetable
Lunch	
Leftover tuna casserole with whole-wheat pasta and peas	1 High-quality meat and seafood
	2 Vegetables
Spicy Hot V8 juice	1 Whole grain
Snack	
Peanut M&M's	1 Sweet
Dinner	
Salmon burger on whole-wheat bread	1 High-quality meat and seafood
Sweet potatoes	2 Vegetables
Peas	1 Other (condiments and sauces)
Beer	
Snack	
Peach	1 Fruit

Sunday

I'm struck by how utterly "normal" my eating looks on this day in particular. Bacon. Peanut butter and jelly. Fajitas. This wasn't my healthiest day of the week, but as normal as it was it still conformed largely to the one rule of the agnostic healthy-eating game and it didn't ruin my chances of achieving the right balance of food types for the whole week. Of course, there are plenty of diet-cult members who would look at this food journal and warn me that I'm headed for an early grave. But I know what to say to them: "Oh, dear, I see they've gotten to you, too."

Breakfast	
Omelet with cheddar cheese, spinach, tomatoes, onions, and capers	1 High-quality meat and seafood
	1 Vegetable
Bacon	1 Fruit
Home-fried potatoes	1 Fried food
Orange juice	1 Low-quality meat and seafood
Coffee	
Lunch	
Split pea soup	2 Vegetables
Old-fashioned peanut butter and 100% raspberry fruit spread sandwich on whole-wheat bread	1 Whole grain
	1 Nuts, seeds, and healthy oils
Spicy Hot V8 juice	½ Fruit
Snack	
Peach	1 Fruit
Dinner	
Chicken and vegetable fajitas with corn tortillas	1 Vegetable
Beer	1 High-quality meat and seafood
Dark chocolate	1 Whole grain
Snack	
Greek yogurt (whole milk) with dried cherries, honey, and Grape Nuts Flakes	1 Dairy
	½ Fruit
	½ Whole grain

Week's Totals

I came fairly close to earning "extra credit" for this week by eating each food type more often than any food type of lesser quality. The only significant departures from "perfect" balance in my diet were a high frequency of whole-grain consumption (which is normal for me because I need my carbs for sports training) and a large number in the "Other Foods" column because of my love of beer. Still, I managed to adhere to the basic rule of eating each "essential" food type more often than any "recommended" food type and each "recommended" food type more often than any "acceptable" food type.

Food Type	Number of Times Eaten This Week
Vegetables	27.5
Fruit	23
Nuts, seeds, and healthy oils	8
High-quality meats and seafood	14
Whole grains	16.5
Dairy	10
Refined grains	2
Other foods	7
Low-quality meats and seafood	1
Sweets	2
Fried foods	1

Further Reading

Chapter 1
Church RM. Emotional reactions of rats to the pain of others. J Comp Physiol Psychol. 1959 Apr;52(2):132-4.

Chang SWC, Gariépy JF,. Platt ML. Nature Neuroscience. Neuronal reference frames for social decisions in primate frontal cortex. 2013 16, 243–250.

Wynn K. Some innate foundations of social and moral cognition. In P. Carruthers, S. Laurence & S. Stich (Eds.), The Innate Mind: Foundations and the Future. 2008. Oxford: Oxford University Press.

Nestle M. What To Eat. North Point Press, 2010.

Marean CW, Bar-Matthews M, Bernatchez J, Fisher E, Goldberg P, Herries AIR, Jacobs Z, Jerardino A, Karkanas P, Minichillo T, Nilssen PJ, Thompson E, Watt I, Williams HM. Early human use of marine resources and pigment in South Africa during the Middle Pleistocene. Nature. 2007 Oct 18;449(7164):905-8.

Chapter 2
Holland LZ. Feasting and Fasting with Lewis & Clark: A Food and Social History of the Early 1800s. Old Yellowstone Publishing, 2003.

Wells S. The Journey of Man: A Genetic Odyssey. Random House, 2012.

Nabhan GP. Why Some Like It Hot: Food, Genes, and Cultural Diversity. Island Press, 2006.

David LA, Maurice CF, Carmody RN, Gootenberg DB, Button JE, Wolfe BE, Ling AV, Devlin AS, Varma Y, Fischbach MA, Biddinger SB, Dutton RJ, Turnbaugh PJ. Diet rapidly and reproducibly alters the human gut microbiome. Nature. 2013 Dec 11."

Groessler ME. Traditional Diet of The Saalish, Kootenai and Pend d'Oreille Indians in North West Montana and Contemporary Diet Recommendations, A Comparison. Diss. Montana State University, Bozeman, 2008.

Allbaugh L. Crete: A Case Study of an Underdeveloped Area. Princeton University Press, 1953.

Shintani TT, Hughes CK, Beckham S, O'Connor HK. Obesity and cardiovascular risk intervention through the ad libitum feeding of traditional Hawaiian diet. Am J Clin Nutr. 1991 Jun;53(6 Suppl):1647S-1651S.

Wall TL, Carr LG, Ehlers CL. Protective association of genetic variation in alcohol dehydrogenase with alcohol dependence in Native American Mission Indians. Am J Psychiatry. 2003 Jan;160(1):41-6.

Zampelas A, Roche H, Knapper JM, Jackson KG, Tornaritis M, Hatzis C, Gibney MJ, Kafatos A, Gould BJ, Wright J, Williams CM. Differences in postprandial lipaemic response between Northern and Southern Europeans. Atherosclerosis. 1998 Jul;139(1):83-93.

Gardener H, Wright CB, Gu Y, Demmer RT, Boden-Albala B, Elkind MS, Sacco RL, Scarmeas N. Mediterranean-style diet and risk of ischemic stroke, myocardial infarction, and vascular death: the Northern Manhattan Study. Am J Clin Nutr. 2011 Dec;94(6):1458-64.

Chapter 3

Bresnahan KA, Arscott SA, Khanna H, Arinaitwe G, Dale J, Tushemereirwe W, Mondloch S, Tanumihardjo JP, De Moura FF, Tanumihardjo SA. Cooking enhances but the degree of ripeness does not affect provitamin A carotenoid bioavailability from bananas in Mongolian gerbils. J Nutr. 2012 Dec;142(12):2097-104.

Zajic L. Raw Food Diet Study. The Iowa Source, Aug 2006.

Wrangham R. Catching Fire: How Cooking Made Us Human. Basic Books, 2010.

Koebnick C, Garcia AL, Dagnelie PC, Strassner C, Lindemans J, Katz N, Leitzmann C, Hoffmann I. Long-Term Consumption of a Raw Food Diet Is Associated with Favorable Serum LDL Cholesterol and Triglycerides but Also with Elevated Plasma Homocysteine and Low Serum HDL Cholesterol in Humans. J Nutr. Oct, 2005 vol. 135 no. 10 2372-2378.

Chapter 4

Wynn JG, Sponheimer M, Kimbel WH, Alemseged Z, Reed K, Bedaso ZK, Wilson JN. Diet of Australopithecus afarensis from the Pliocene Hadar Formation, Ethiopia. Proc Natl Acad Sci.

Cerling TE, Manthi FK, Mbua EN, Leakey LN, Leakey MG, Leakey RE, Brown FH, Grine FE, Hart JA, Kaleme P, Roche H, Uno KT, Wood BA. Stable isotope-based diet reconstructions of Turkana Basin hominins. Proc Natl Acad Sci.

Cerling TE, Chritz KL, Jablonski NG, Leakey MG, Manthi FK. Diet of Theropithecus from 4 to 1 Ma in Kenya. Proc Natl Acad Sci.

Sponheimer M, Alemseged Z, Cerling TE, Grine FE, Kimbel WH, Leakey MG, Lee-Thorp JA, Manthi FK, Reed KE, Wood BA, Wynn JG. Isotopic evidence of early hominin diets. Proc Natl Acad Sci.

Pan A, Sun Q, Bernstein AM, Schulze MB, Manson JE, Stampfer MJ, Willett WC, Hu FB. Red meat consumption and mortality: results from 2 prospective cohort studies. Arch Intern Med. 2012 Apr 9;172(7):555-63.

Elwood PC, Pickering JE, Givens DI, Gallacher JE. Lipids. The consumption of milk and dairy foods and the incidence of vascular disease and diabetes: an overview of the evidence. 2010 Oct;45(10):925-39.

Schatzkin A, Mouw T, Park Y, Subar AF, Kipnis V, Hollenbeck A, Leitzmann MF, Thompson FE. Dietary fiber and whole-grain consumption in relation to colorectal cancer in the NIH-AARP Diet and Health Study. Am J Clin Nutr. 2007 May;85(5):1353-60.

Bouchenak M, Lamri-Senhadji M. Nutritional quality of legumes, and their role in cardiometabolic risk prevention: a review. J Med Food. 2013 Mar; 16(3):185-98.

Gerbault P, Liebert A, Itan Y, Powell A, Currat M, Burger J, Swallow DM, Thomas MG. Evolution of lactase persistence: an example of human niche construction. Philos Trans R Soc Lond B Biol Sci. 2011 Mar 27;366(1566):863-77.

Perry GH, Dominy NJ, Claw KG, Lee AS, Fiegler H, Redon R, Werner J, Villanea FA, Mountain JL, Misra R, Carter NP, Lee C, Stone AC. Diet and the evolution of human amylase gene copy number variation. Nat Genet. 2007 Oct;39(10):1256-60.

Squires BT. Human salivary amylase secretion in relation to diet. J Physiol. 1953;119:153–156.

Robinson E, Blissett J, Higgs S. Social influences on eating: implications for nutritional interventions. Nutr Res Rev. 2013 Dec;26(2):166-76.

Trexler, E. Paleolithic diet is associated with unfavorable changes to blood lipids in healthy subjects. (Unpublished)

Chapter 5

Jebb SA, Ahern AL, Olson AD, Aston LM, Holzapfel C, Stoll J, Amann-Gassner U, Simpson AE, Fuller NR, Pearson S, Lau NS, Mander AP, Hauner H, Caterson ID. Primary care referral to a commercial provider for weight loss treatment versus standard care: a randomised controlled trial. Lancet. 2011 Oct 22;378(9801):1485-92.

Lowe MR, Kral TV, Miller-Kovach K. Weight-loss maintenance 1, 2 and 5 years after successful completion of a weight-loss programme. Br J Nutr. 2008 Apr;99(4):925-30.

Butryn ML, Phelan S, Hill JO, Wing RR. Consistent self-monitoring of weight: a key component of successful weight loss maintenance. Obesity (Silver Spring). 2007 Dec;15(12):3091-6.

Raynor HA, Jeffery RW, Phelan S, Hill JO, Wing RR. Amount of food group variety consumed in the diet and long-term weight loss maintenance. Obes Res. 2005 May;13(5):883-90.

Gorin AA, Phelan S, Hill JO, Wing RR. Promoting long-term weight control: does dieting consistency matter? Int J Obes Relat Metab Disord. 2004 Feb;28(2):278-81.

Yanovski JA, Yanovski SZ, Sovik KN, Nguyen TT, O'Neil PM, Sebring NG. A prospective study of holiday weight gain. N Engl J Med. 2000 Mar 23;342(12):861-7.

Racette SB, Weiss EP, Schechtman KB, Steger-May K, Villareal DT, Obert KA, Holloszy JO. 2008. Influence of Weekend Lifestyle Patterns on Body Weight. Obesity 16(8):1826–30.

Catenacci VA, Grunwald GK, Ingebrigtsen JP, Jakicic JM, McDermott MD, Phelan S, Wing RR, Hill JO, Wyatt HR. Physical activity patterns using accelerometry in the National Weight Control Registry. Obesity (Silver Spring). 2011 Jun;19(6):1163-70.

Le DS, Pannacciulli N, Chen K, Salbe AD, Del Parigi A, Hill JO, Wing RR, Reiman EM, Krakoff J. Less activation in the left dorsolateral prefrontal cortex in the reanalysis of the response to a meal in obese than in lean women and its association with successful weight loss. Am J Clin Nutr. 2007 Sep;86(3):573-9.

Mischel W, Ayduk O, Berman MG, Casey BJ, Gotlib IH, Jonides J, Kross E, Teslovich T, Wilson NL, Zayas V, Shoda Y. "Willpower" over the life span: decomposing self-regulation. Soc Cogn Affect Neurosci. 2011 Apr;6(2):252-6.

Baumeister RF, Tierney J. Willpower: Rediscovering the Greatest Human Strength. 2012, Penguin Books.

Klem ML, Wing RR, McGuire MT, Seagle HM, Hill JO. A descriptive study of individuals successful at long-term maintenance of substantial weight loss. Am J Clin Nutr. 1997 Aug;66(2):239-46.

Ohsiek S, Williams M. Psychological factors influencing weight loss maintenance: an integrative literature review. J Am Acad Nurse Pract. 2011 Nov;23(11):592-601.

Carnell S, Gibson C, Benson L, Ochner CN, Geliebter A. Neuroimaging and obesity: current knowledge and future directions. Obes Rev. 2012 Jan;13(1):43-56.

Food Addiction? Special issue of Biological Psychiatry. Vol. 73, No. 9; May 1, 2013.

Jeffery RW. Financial incentives and weight control. Prev Med. 2012 Nov;55 Suppl:S61-7.

Chapter 6

Westman EC. Is dietary carbohydrate essential for human nutrition? *Am J Clin Nutr* May 2002 vol. 75 no. 5 951-953.

Gandy JJ, Snyman JR, van Rensburg CE. Randomized, parallel-group, double-blind, controlled study to evaluate the efficacy and safety of carbohydrate-derived fulvic acid in topical treatment of eczema. Clin Cosmet Investig Dermatol. 2011;4:145-8.

Udani JK, Singh BB, Singh VJ, Barrett ML. Effects of Açai (Euterpe oleracea Mart.) berry preparation on metabolic parameters in a healthy overweight population: a pilot study. Nutr J 2011 May 12;10:45.

Chapter 7

Reader J. Potato: A History of the Propitious Esculent. Yale University Press, 2011.

Hindhede M. Vegetarian experiment with a population of 3 million. JAMA. Feb. 7. 1920, Volume 74, Number 6.

Kon SK, Klein A. The value of whole potato in human nutrition. Biochem J. 1928; 22(1): 258–260

Gordon ES, Marshall G, Chosy GJ. A new concept in the treatment of obesity. JAMA 1963 Oct 5—pp. 156-163—Vol. 186, No. 1.

Holt SH, Miller JC, Petocz P, Farmakalidis E. A satiety index of common foods. Eur J Clin Nutr. 1995 Sep;49(9):675-90.

Drewnowski A, Rehm CD. Vegetable cost metrics show that potatoes and beans provide most nutrients per penny. PLoS One. 2013 May 15;8(5):e63277.

Chapter 8
Church TS, Martin CK, Thompson AM, Earnest CP, Mikus CR, Blair SN. Changes in weight, waist circumference and compensatory responses with different doses of exercise among sedentary, overweight postmenopausal women. PLoS One. 2009;4(2):e4515.

Hopkins M, Blundell JE, King NA. Individual variability in compensatory eating following acute exercise in overweight and obese women. Br J Sports Med. 2013 May 10.

Burke LM. Nutritional practices of male and female endurance athletes. Sports Med. 2001;31(7):521-32.

Teixeira A, Müller L, dos Santos AA, Reckziegel P, Emanuelli T, Rocha JB, Bürger ME. Beneficial effects of gradual intense exercise in tissues of rats fed with a diet deficient in vitamins and minerals: a pilot study. Nutrition. 2009 May;25(5):590-6.

Christensen DL, Jakobsen J, Friis H. Vitamin and mineral intake of twelve adolescent male Kalenjin runners in western Kenya. East Afr Med J. 2005 Dec;82(12):637-42.

Mestek ML, Plaisance EP, Ratcliff LA, Taylor JK, Wee SO, Grandjean PW. Aerobic exercise and postprandial lipemia in men with the metabolic syndrome. Med Sci Sports Exerc. 2008 Dec;40(12):2105-11.

Fontana L, Meyer TE, Klein S, Holloszy JO. Long-term low-calorie low-protein vegan diet and endurance exercise are associated with low cardiometabolic risk. Rejuvenation Res. 2007 Jun;10(2):225-34.

Sui X, LaMonte MJ, Laditka JN, Hardwin JW, Chase N, Hooker SP, Blair SN. Cardiorespiratory fitness and adiposity as mortality predictors in older adults. JAMA. 2007 Dec 5;298(21):2507-16.

Nieman DC, Sherman KM, Arabatzis K, et al. Hematological,anthropometric, and metabolic comparisons between vegetarian and nonvegetarian elderly women. Int J Sports Med 1989;10:243–50.

Koutsari C, Hardman AE. Exercise prevents the augmentation of postprandial lipaemia attributable to a low-fat high-carbohydrate diet. Br J Nutr. 2001 Aug;86(2):197-205.

Legaz-Arrese A, Kinfu H, Munguía-Izquierdo D, Carranza-Garcia LE, Calderón FJ. Basic physiological measures determine fitness and are associated with running performance in elite young male and female Ethiopian runners. J Sports Med Phys Fitness. 2009 Dec;49(4):358-63.

Chapter 9
Kawachi I, Willett WC, Colditz GA, Stampfer MJ, Speizer FE. A prospective study of coffee drinking and suicide in women. Arch Intern Med. 1996 Mar 11;156(5):521-5.

Lucas M, Mirzaei F, Pan A, Okereke OI, Willett WC, O'Reilly ÉJ, Koenen K, Ascherio A. Coffee, caffeine, and risk of depression among women. Arch Intern Med. 2011 Sep 26;171(17):1571-8.

Freedman ND, Park Y, Abnet CC, Hollenbeck AR, Sinha R. Association of coffee drinking with total and cause-specific mortality. N Engl J Med. 2012 May 17;366(20):1891-904.

Cano-Marquina A, Tarín JJ, Cano A. The impact of coffee on health. Maturitas. 2013 May;75(1):7-21.

Duncan MJ, Oxford SW. Acute caffeine ingestion enhances performance and dampens muscle pain following resistance exercise to failure. J Sports Med Phys Fitness. 2012 Jun;52(3):280-5.

Astorino TA, Cottrell T, Talhami Lozano A, Aburto-Pratt K, Duhon J. Effect of caffeine on RPE and perceptions of pain, arousal, and pleasure/displeasure during a cycling time trial in endurance trained and active men. Physiol Behav. 2012 May 15;106(2):211-7.

Rein D, Paglieroni TG, Wun T, Pearson DA, Schmitz HH, Gosselin R, Keen CL. Cocoa inhibits platelet activation and function. Am J Clin Nutr. 2000 Jul;72(1):30-5.

Ding EL, Hutfless SM, Ding X, Girotra S. Chocolate and prevention of cardiovascular disease: a systematic review. Nutr Metab (Lond). 2006 Jan 3;3:2.

Katz DL, Doughty K, Ali A. Cocoa and chocolate in human health and disease. Antioxid Redox Signal. 2011 Nov 15;15(10):2779-811.

Golomb BA, Koperski S, White HL. Association between more frequent chocolate consumption and lower body mass index. Arch Intern Med. 2012 Mar 26;172(6):519-21.

Parker G, Parker I, Brotchie H. Mood state effects of chocolate. J Affect Disord. 2006 Jun;92(2-3):149-59.

Klatsky AL. Alcohol and cardiovascular health. *Integr. Comp. Biol.* (2004) 44 (4): 324-328.

Baur JA, Pearson KJ, Price NL, Jamieson HA, Lerin C, Kalra A, Prabhu VV, Allard JS, Lopez-Lluch G, Lewis K, Pistell PJ, Poosala S, Becker KG, Boss O, Gwinn D, Wang M, Ramaswamy S, Fishbein KW, Spencer RG, Lakatta EG, Le Couteur D, Shaw RJ, Navas P, Puigserver P, Ingram DK, de Cabo R, Sinclair DA. Resveratrol improves health and survival of mice on a high-calorie diet. Nature. 2006 Nov 16;444(7117):337-42.

Koppes LL, Dekker JM, Hendriks HF, Bouter LM, Heine RJ. Moderate alcohol consumption lowers the risk of type 2 diabetes: a meta-analysis of prospective observational studies. Diabetes Care. 2005 Mar;28(3):719-25.

Stewart SH, Mainous AG 3rd, Gilbert G. Relation between alcohol consumption and C-reactive protein levels in the adult US population. J Am Board Fam Pract. 2002 Nov-Dec;15(6):437-42.

Marmot MG, Shipley MJ, Rose G, Thomas BJ. Alcohol and mortality: a u-shaped curve. Lancet. 1981 Mar 14;1(8220 Pt 1):580-3.

Tepper BJ, Ullrich NV. Influence of genetic taste sensitivity to 6-n-propylthiouracil (PROP), dietary restraint and disinhibition on body mass index in middle-aged women. Physiol Behav. 2002 Mar;75(3):305-12.

Shirai K, Iso H, Ohira T, Ikeda A, Noda H, Honjo K, Inoue M, Tsugane S; Japan Public Health Center-Based Study Group. Perceived level of life enjoyment and risks of cardiovascular disease incidence and mortality: the Japan public health center-based study. Circulation. 2009 Sep 15;120(11):956-63.

Chapter 10
Cade R, Spooner G, Schlein E, Pickering M, Dean R. J Sports Med Phys Fitness. Effect of fluid, electrolyte, and glucose replacement during exercise on performance, body temperature, rate of sweat loss, and compositional changes of extracellular fluid. 1972 Sep;12(3):150-6.

Hew TD, Chorley JN, Cianca JC, Divine JG. The incidence, risk factors, and clinical manifestations of hyponatremia in marathon runners. Clin J Sport Med. 2003 Jan;13(1):41-7.

Glover B, Glover SF. The Competitive Runner's Handbook. Penguin Books, 1999.

Batmanghelidj F. Your Body's Many Cries for Water. Global Health Solutions, 1992.

Noakes T. Waterlogged: The Serious Problem of Overhydration in Endurance Sports. Human Kinetics, 2012.

Wyndham CH, Strydom NB. The danger of inadequate water intake during marathon running. S Afr Med J. 1969 Jul 19;43(29):893-6.

Daries HN, Noakes TD, Dennis SC. Effect of fluid intake volume on 2-h running performances in a 25 degrees C environment. Med Sci Sports Exerc. 2000 Oct;32(10):1783-9.

Schulze MB, Manson JE, Ludwig DS, Colditz GA, Stampfer MJ, Willett WC, Hu FB. Sugar-sweetened beverages, weight gain, and incidence of type 2 diabetes in young and middle-aged women. JAMA. 2004;292:927-934.

Hu FB, Malik VS. Sugar-sweetened beverages and risk of obesity and type 2 diabetes: epidemiologic evidence. Physiol Behav. 2010 Apr 26;100(1):47-54.

Jeukendrup A, Brouns F, Wagenmakers AJ, Saris WH. Carbohydrate-electrolyte feedings improve 1 h time trial cycling performance. Int J Sports Med. 1997 Feb;18(2):125-9.

Smith JW, Zachwieja JJ, Péronnet F, Passe DH, Massicotte D, Lavoie C, Pascoe DD. Fuel selection and cycling endurance performance with ingestion of [13C]glucose: evidence for a carbohydrate dose response. J Appl Physiol. 2010 Jun;108(6):1520-9.

Stannard SR, Hawke EJ, Schnell N. The effect of galactose supplementation on endurance cycling performance. Eur J Clin Nutr. 2009 Feb;63(2):209-14.

Jeukendrup AE, Vet-Joop K, Sturk A, Stegen JH, Senden J, Saris WH, Wagenmakers AJ. Relationship between gastro-intestinal complaints and endotoxaemia, cytokine release and the acute-phase reaction during and after a long-distance triathlon in highly trained men. Clin Sci (Lond). 2000 Jan;98(1):47-55.

Peternelj TT, Coombes JS. Sports Med. Antioxidant supplementation during exercise training: beneficial or detrimental? 2011 Dec 1;41(12):1043-69.

Chapter 11
Hartman AL, Rubenstein JE, Kossoff EH. Intermittent fasting: A "new" historical strategy for controlling seizures? Epilepsy Res. 2013 May;104(3):275-9.

Kjeldsen-Kragh J, Haugen M, Borchgrevink CF, Laerum E, Eek M, Mowinkel P, Hovi K, Førre O. Controlled trial of fasting and one-year vegetarian diet in rheumatoid arthritis. Lancet. 1991 Oct 12;338(8772):899-902.

Lee C, Raffaghello L, Brandhorst S, Safdie FM, Bianchi G, Martin-Montalvo A, Pistoia V, Wei M, Hwang S, Merlino A, Emionite L, de Cabo R, Longo VD. Fasting cycles retard growth of tumors and sensitize a range of cancer cell types to chemotherapy. Sci Transl Med. 2012 Mar 7;4(124):124ra27.

Lee C, Raffaghello L, Longo VD. Starvation, detoxification, and multidrug resistance in cancer therapy. Drug Resist Updat. 2012 Feb-Apr;15(1-2):114-22.

Raffaghello L, Safdie F, Bianchi G, Dorff T, Fontana L, Longo VD. Fasting and differential chemotherapy protection in patients. Cell Cycle. 2010 Nov 15;9(22):4474-6.

Harvie MN, Pegington M, Mattson MP, Frystyk J, Dillon B, Evans G, Cuzick J, Jebb SA, Martin B, Cutler RG, Son TG, Maudsley S, Carlson OD, Egan JM, Flyvbjerg A, Howell A. Int J Obes (Lond). The effects of intermittent or continuous energy restriction on weight loss and metabolic disease risk markers: a randomized trial in young overweight women. 2011 May;35(5):714-27.

McCay C, Crowell M, Maynard L. (1935). The effect of retarded growth upon the length of life and upon ultimate size. J Nutr 10:63-79.

Mohan PF, Rao BS. Adaptation to underfeeding in growing rats. Effect of energy restriction at two dietary protein levels on growth, feed efficiency, basal metabolism and body composition. J Nutr. 1983 Jan;113(1):79-85.

Calabrese V, Cornelius C, Cuzzocrea S, Iavicoli I, Rizzarelli E, Calabrese EJ. Hormesis, cellular stress response and vitagenes as critical determinants in aging and longevity. Mol Aspects Med. 2011 Aug;32(4-6):279-304.

Wang Y, Lawler D, Larson B, Ramadan Z, Kochhar S, Holmes E, Nicholson JK. Metabonomic investigations of aging and caloric restriction in a life-long dog study. J Proteome Res. 2007 May;6(5):1846-54.

Colman RJ, Anderson RM, Johnson SC, Kastman EK, Kosmatka KJ, Beasley TM, Allison DB, Cruzen C, Simmons HA, Kemnitz JW, Weindruch R. Caloric restriction delays disease onset and mortality in rhesus monkeys. Science. 2009 Jul 10;325(5937):201-4.

Mattison JA, Roth GS, Beasley TM, Tilmont EM, Handy AM, Herbert RL, Longo DL, Allison DB, Young JE, Bryant M, Barnard D, Ward WF, Qi W, Ingram DK, de Cabo R. Impact of caloric restriction on health and survival in rhesus monkeys from the NIA study. Nature. 2012 Sep 13;489(7415):318-21.

Chapter 12
Ludvigsson JF, Rubio-Tapia A, van Dyke CT, Melton LJ 3rd, Zinsmeister AR, Lahr BD, Murray JA. Increasing incidence of celiac disease in a North American population. Am J Gastroenterol. 2013 May;108(5):818-24.

Sapone A, Lammers KM, Casolaro V, Cammarota M, Giuliano MT, De Rosa M, Stefanile R, Mazzarella G, Tolone C, Russo MI, Esposito P, Ferraraccio F, Cartenì M, Riegler G, de Magistris L, Fasano A. Divergence of gut permeability and mucosal immune gene expression in two gluten-associated conditions: celiac disease and gluten sensitivity. BMC Med. 2011 Mar 9;9:23.

Biesiekierski JR, Peters SL, Newnham ED, Rosella O, Muir JG, Gibson PR. No Effects of Gluten in Patients with Self-Reported Non-Celiac Gluten Sensitivity Following Dietary Reduction of Low-Fermentable, Poorly-Absorbed, Short-Chain Carbohydrates. Gastroenterology. 2013 May 3. doi:pii: S0016-5085(13)00702-6.

Di Sabatino A, Corazza GR. Nonceliac gluten sensitivity: sense of sensibility? Ann Intern Med. 2012 Feb 21;156(4):309-11.

Chang PP, Ford DE, Meoni LA, Wang NY, Klag MJ. Anger in young men and subsequent premature cardiovascular disease: the precursors study. Arch Intern Med. 2002 Apr 22;162(8):901-6.

Steptoe A, Shankar A, Demakakos P, Wardle J. Social isolation, loneliness, and all-cause mortality in older men and women. Proc Natl Acad Sci U S A. 2013 Apr 9;110(15):5797-801.

Dube SR, Fairweather D, Pearson WS, Felitti VJ, Andra RF, Croft JB. Cumulative childhood stress and autoimmune diseases in adults. Psychosom Med. 2009 Feb;71(2):243-50.

Lederbogen F, Kirsch P, Haddad L, Streit F, Tost H, Schuch P, Wüst S, Pruessner JC, Rietschel M, Deuschle M, Meyer-Lindenberg A. City living and urban upbringing affect neural social stress processing in humans. Nature. Jun 22;474(7352):498-501.

Krabbendam L, van Os J. Schizophrenia and urbanicity: a major environmental influence--conditional on genetic risk. Schizophr Bull. 2005 Oct;31(4):795-9. Epub 2005 Sep 8.

Bobrow-Strain A. White Bread: A Social History of the Store-Bought Loaf. Beacon Press, 2013.

Chapter 13
Liebig J. (1842/1964). Animal Chemistry or Organic Chemistry in its Application to Physiology and Pathology. New York, Johnson Reprint Corporation.

Carpenter K. (1994). Protein and Energy: A Study of Changing Ideas in Nutrition. Cambridge, Cambridge University Press.

Kraut H, Muller EA, Muller-Wecker H. Dependence of muscular training and protein deposit upon protein uptake and protein content in the body. Biochem Z. 1953;324(4):280-94.

Fox EA, McDaniel JL, Breitbach AP, Weiss EP. Perceived protein needs and measured protein intake in collegiate male athletes: an observational study. J Int Soc Sports Nutr. 2011 Jun 21;8:9.

Lemon PW, Tarnopolsky MA, MacDougall JD, Atkinson SA. Protein requirements and muscle mass/strength changes during intensive training in novice bodybuilders. J Appl Physiol. 1992 Aug;73(2):767-75.

Hartman JW, Moore DR, Phillips SM. Appl Physiol Nutr Metab. Resistance training reduces whole-body protein turnover and improves net protein retention in untrained young males. 2006 Oct;31(5):557-64.

Harris RC, Söderlund K, Hultman E. Elevation of creatine in resting and exercised muscle of normal subjects by creatine supplementation. Clin Sci (Lond). 1992 Sep;83(3):367-74.

Greenhaff PL, Casey A, Short AH, Harris R, Soderlund K, Hultman E. Influence of oral creatine supplementation of muscle torque during repeated bouts of maximal voluntary exercise in man. Clin Sci (Lond). 1993 May;84(5):565-71.

Gualano B, Roschel H, Lancha-Jr AH, Brightbill CE, Rawson ES. Amino Acids. 2012 Aug;43(2):519-29. Amino Acids. 2012 Aug;43(2):519-29.

Nissen S, Sharp R, Ray M, Rathmacher JA, Rice D, Fuller JC Jr, Connelly AS, Abumrad N. Effect of leucine metabolite beta-hydroxy-beta-methylbutyrate on muscle metabolism during resistance-exercise training. J Appl Physiol. 1996 Nov;81(5):2095-104.

Rowlands DS, Thomson JS. Effects of beta-hydroxy-beta-methylbutyrate supplementation during resistance training on strength, body composition, and muscle damage in trained and untrained young men: a meta-analysis. J Strength Cond Res. 2009 May;23(3):836-46.

Chapter 14

Ryan MF, Grada CO, Morris C, Segurado R, Walsh MC, Gibney ER, Brennan L, Roche HM, Gibney MJ. Within-person variation in the postprandial lipemic response of healthy adults. Am J Clin Nutr. 2013 Feb;97(2):261-7.

Pusztai A. Dietary lectins are metabolic signals for the gut and modulate immune and hormone functions. Eur J Clin Nutr. 1993 Oct;47(10):691-9.

Trumbo P, Schlicker S, Yates AA, Poos M; Food and Nutrition Board of the Institute of Medicine, The National Academies. Dietary reference intakes for energy, carbohydrate, fiber, fat, fatty acids, cholesterol, protein and amino acids. J Am Diet Assoc. 2002 Nov;102(11):1621-30.

Grallert H, Sedlmeier EM, Huth C, Kolz M, Heid IM, Meisinger C, Herder C, Strassburger K, Gehringer A, Haak M, Giani G, Kronenberg F, Wichmann HE, Adamski J, Paulweber B, Illig T, Rathmann W. APOA5 gene variation modulates the effects of dietary fat intake on body mass index and obesity risk in the Framingham Heart Study. J Mol Med (Berl). 2007 Feb;85(2):119-28.

Zeisel SH. Nutritional genomics: defining the dietary requirement and effects of choline. J Nutr. 2011 Mar;141(3):531-4.

Henríquez Sánchez P, Ruano C, de Irala J, Ruiz-Canela M, Martínez-González MA, Sánchez-Villegas A. Adherence to the Mediterranean diet and quality of life in the SUN Project. ur J Clin Nutr. 2012 Mar;66(3):360-8.

Chapter 15

Slavin JL, Lloyd B. Health benefits of fruits and vegetables. Adv Nutr. 2012 Jul 1;3(4):506-16.

Liu RH. Health benefit of fruit and vegetables are from additive and synergistic combinations of phytochemicals. Am J Clin Nutr. 2003 Sept;78(3):517S-520S.

Flores-Mateo G, Rojas-Rueda D, Basora J, Ros E, Salas-Salvadó J. Nut intake and adiposity: meta-analysis of clinical trials. Am J Clin Nutr. 2013 Apr 17.

Ying B, Han J, Hu FB, Giovannucci EL, Stampfer MJ, Willett WC, Fuchs CS. Association of nut consumption with total and cause-specific mortality. N Engl J Med 2013; 369:2001-2011.

Tan ZS, Harris WS, Beiser AS, Au R, Himali JJ, Debette S, Pikula A, Decarli C, Wolf PA, Vasan RS, Robins SJ, Seshadri S. Neurology. 2012 Feb 28;78(9):658-64. Red blood cell omega-3 fatty acid levels and markers of accelerated brain aging.

Vander Wal JS, Gupta A, Khosla P, Dhurandhar NV. Egg breakfast enhances weight loss. Int J Obes (Lond). 2008 Oct;32(10):1545-51.

Lefevre M, Jonnalagadda S. Effect of whole grains on markers of subclinical inflammation. Nutr Rev. 2012 Jul;70(7):387-96.

Ellwood PC, Pickering JE, Givens DI, Gallacher JE. The consumption of milk and dairy foods and the incidence of vascular disease and diabetes: an overview of the evidence. Lipids. 2010 Oct;45(10):925-39.

Sinha R, Cross AJ, Graubard BI, Leitzmann MF, Schatzkin A. Meat intake and mortality: a prospective study of over half a million people. Arch Intern Med. 2009 Mar 23;169(6):562-71.

Guallar-Castillón P, Rodríguez-Artalejo F, Fornés NS, Banegas JR, Etxezarreta PA, Ardanaz E, Barricarte A, Chirlaque MD, Iraeta MD, Larrañaga NL, Losada A, Mendez M, Martínez C, Quirós JR, Navarro C, Jakszyn P, Sánchez MJ, Tormo MJ, González CA. Intake of fried foods is associated with obesity in the cohort of Spanish adults from the European Prospective Investigation into Cancer and Nutrition. Am J Clin Nutr. 2007 Jul;86(1):198-205.

El-Sayyad HI, El-Gammal HL, Habak LA, Abdel-Galil HM, Fernando A, Gaur RL, Ouhtit A. Structural and ultrastructural evidence of neurotoxic effects of fried potato chips on rat postnatal development. Nutrition. 2011 Oct;27(10):1066-75.

Feijó Fde M, Ballard CR, Foletto KC, Batista BA, Neves AM, Ribeiro MF, Bertoluci MC. Saccharin and aspartame, compared with sucrose, induce greater weight gain in adult Wistar rats, at similar total caloric intake levels. Appetite. 2013 Jan;60(1):203-7.

Acknowledgments

I wish to express my heartfelt gratitude to the many people who helped me with this book: to Brandy Alles, Anthony Famiglietti, Laurie Fitzgerald, Kara Goucher, Lucy Gustafson, Bernie Freeman, Brian MacKenzie, and John Romaniello for sharing—and permitting me to share—their stories; to Nataki Fitzgerald, Tom Fitzgerald, and John Berardi for reading and commenting on early versions of select chapters; to Michelle Lacey for teaching me about epigenetics; to Steve Delmonte for bringing my cartoon concepts to life; to Phil Gaskill, Maria Fernandez, and the team at FaceOut Studio for transforming my messy Word files into a polished and attractive finished product; to Chuck Monroe of Gold Dust Publicity for creating a buzz; to Linda Konner for championing my original vision; and to Jessica Case and Claiborne Hancock for giving me the opportunity, the freedom, and the support to make the vision real.